To
John W. Kimball

CONTENTS

LIST OF TOPICS & ILLUSTRATIONS

Text: One page of text is devoted to each of the following topics. *Illustrations are listed in italics.*

PREFACE

An Illustrated Review of Anatomy and Physiology is a series of ten books written to help students effectively review the structure and function of the human body. Each book in the series is devoted to a different body system.

My objective in writing these books is to make very complex subjects accessible and unthreatening by presenting material in manageable size bits (one topic per page) with clear, simple illustrations to assist the many students who are primarily visual learners. Designed to supplement established texts, they may be used as a student aid to jog the memory, to quickly recall the essentials of each major topic, and to practice naming structures in preparation for exams.

INNOVATIVE FEATURES OF THE BOOK

(1) Each major topic is confined to one page of text.

A unique feature of this book is that each topic is confined to one page and the material is presented in outline form with the key terms in boldface or italic typeface. This makes it easy to scan quickly the major points of any given topic. The student can easily get an overview of the topic and then zero in on a particular point that needs clarification.

(2) Each page of text has an illustration on the facing page.

Because each page of text has its illustration on the facing page, there is no need to flip through the book looking for the illustration that is referred to in the text ("see Figure X on page xx"). The purpose of the illustration is to clarify a central idea discussed in the text. The images are simple and clear, the lines are bold, and the labels are in a large type. Each illustration deals with a well-defined concept, allowing for a more focused study.

> ***PHYSIOLOGY TOPICS*** (1 text page : 1 illustration)
> Each main topic in physiology is limited to one page of text with one supporting illustration on the facing page.

ANATOMY TOPICS (1 text page : several illustrations)
For complex anatomical structures a good illustration is more valuable than words. So, for topics dealing with anatomy, there are often several illustrations for one text topic.

(3) *Unlabeled illustrations have been included.*
In Part II, all illustrations have been repeated without their labels. This allows a student to test his or her visual knowledge of the basic concepts.

(4) *A Pronunciation Guide has been included.*
Phonetic spellings of unfamiliar terms are listed in a separate section, unlike other textbooks where they are usually found in the glossary or spread throughout the text. The student may use this guide for pronunciation drill or as a quick review of basic vocabulary.

(5) *A glossary has been included.*
Most textbooks have glossaries that include terms for all of the systems of the body. It is convenient to have all of the key terms for one system in a single glossary.

ACKNOWLEDGMENTS

I would like to thank the reviewers of the manuscript for this book who carefully critiqued the text and illustrations for their effectiveness: William Kleinelp, Middlesex County College; and Robert Smith, University of Missouri, St. Louis, and St. Louis Community College, Forest Park. Their help and advice are greatly appreciated. Kay Petronio is to be commended for her handsome cover design and Bob Cooper has my gratitude for keeping the production moving smoothly. Finally, I am greatly indebted to my editor Bonnie Roesch for her willingness to try a new idea, and for her support throughout this project. I invite students and instructors to send any comments and suggestions for enhancements or changes to this book to me, in care of HarperCollins, so that future editions can continue to meet your needs.

Glenn Bastian

1 Introduction

INTRODUCTION / Overview

PATHOGENS

Organism An organism is any living thing, plant or animal.

Pathogen A pathogen is a disease-causing organism.

Microbe (microorganism) A microbe or microorganism is any microscopic organism (too small to be seen without a microscope). Those of medical interest include bacteria, viruses, fungi, and protozoa (one-celled animals).

Parasite A parasite is a plant or animal that lives upon or inside another organism (its host) and causes damage. The terms pathogenic and parasitic are synonyms; both mean disease-causing.

Most pathogens belong to one of the following types of organisms:

Bacteria
Viruses
Fungi
Protozoa
Parasitic Worms

NONSPECIFIC RESISTANCE

The First Line of Defense The skin and mucous membranes provide a physical barrier that blocks the entrance of most pathogens into the body. Chemical secretions such as mucus, acids, and hydrolytic enzymes trap and kill many microbes before they can enter the body tissues.

Inflammatory Response If pathogenic organisms get past the external barriers to infection, they enter the tissue spaces and cause damage to the cells. The body's response to tissue damage is called the inflammatory response. It is called the inflammatory response because the infected region of the body becomes inflamed (swollen, red, warm, and sore).   There is increased blood flow to the area, the capillaries become more permeable, and phagocytic white blood cells migrate to the region to ingest the pathogenic organisms. The response is the same regardless of the kind of pathogen, so it is called a nonspecific response.

LYMPHATIC TISSUES

Lymphatic tissue is a specialized form of reticular connective tissue that contains large numbers of lymphocytes (a type of white blood cell). The main organs that contain lymphatic tissue are the red bone marrow, thymus, lymph nodes, and spleen. Lymphatic tissue is also present in the mucous membranes that line the tracts of the body (gastrointestinal, respiratory, urinary, and reproductive tracts).

IMMUNE RESPONSES (Specific Responses)

Immune responses provide protection against specific disease-causing agents; they are responsible for the type of resistance called immunity. Immune responses are mediated by lymphocytes (B cells and T cells).

There are two basic types of immunity :
> *(1) Cell-Mediated Immunity (CMI)* Effective against *intracellular* pathogens.
>   Also called *Cellular Immunity*.
> *(2) Antibody-Mediated Immunity (AMI)* Effective against *extracellular* pathogens.
>   Also called *Humoral Immunity*.

INFECTIONS
Infections arise when pathogens enter the body and multiply.

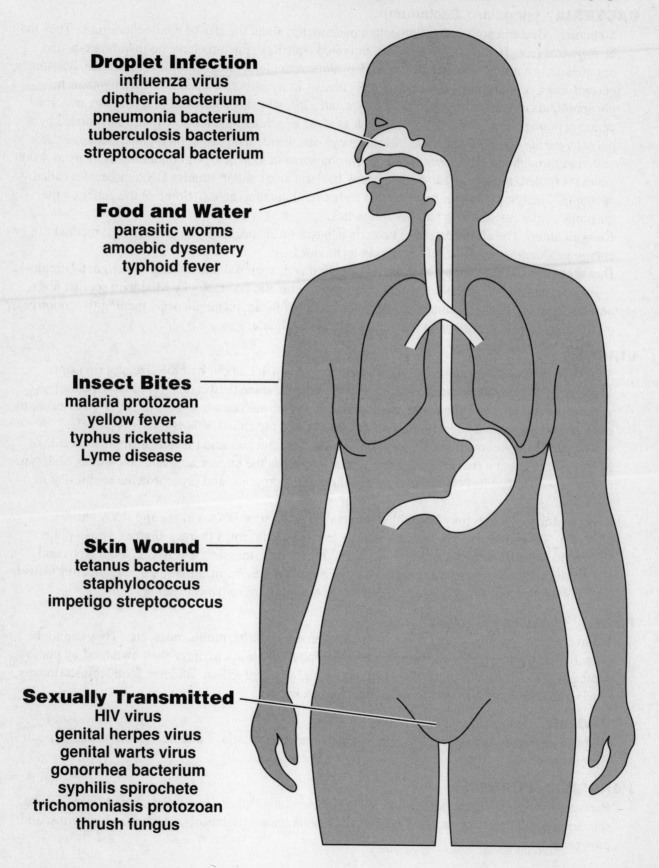

Droplet Infection
influenza virus
diptheria bacterium
pneumonia bacterium
tuberculosis bacterium
streptococcal bacterium

Food and Water
parasitic worms
amoebic dysentery
typhoid fever

Insect Bites
malaria protozoan
yellow fever
typhus rickettsia
Lyme disease

Skin Wound
tetanus bacterium
staphylococcus
impetigo streptococcus

Sexually Transmitted
HIV virus
genital herpes virus
genital warts virus
gonorrhea bacterium
syphilis spirochete
trichomoniasis protozoan
thrush fungus

INTRODUCTION / Pathogens

BACTERIA   (singular : Bacterium)

Structure   Bacteria are 1 to 2 micrometers in diameter, about the size of a mitochondrion. They may be spherical (cocci), rod-shaped (bacilli), or coiled (spirilla). Bacteria have no membrane-bound organelles : no nucleus, mitochondria, endoplasmic reticulum, Golgi complex, centrioles, lysosomes, peroxisomes, or inclusions. A bacterial cell consists of a *plasma membrane*, which contains no phospholipids or cholesterol, surrounded by a *cell wall*, which is composed of a complex material called peptidoglycan. Some cell walls, such as those of virulent pneumococci, are surrounded by a *polysaccharide capsule*, which inhibits phagocytosis. Inside the plasma membrane *ribosomes* are scattered throughout the cytosol. A single chromosome (a loop of DNA containing as many as 4,000 genes) is folded into a *"nuclear body"*. Many bacteria also contain smaller DNA molecules called *plasmids*, which may contain between two and several hundred genes. Some of the genes on the plasmids confer resistance to various antibiotics.

Classification   The classification of bacteria is based on shape, ability to form spores, method of energy production, and reaction to staining techniques.

Diseases   Diseases caused by bacteria include diptheria, bacterial pneumonia, impetigo, tuberculosis, syphilis, typhus fever, typhoid fever, scarlet fever, rheumatic fever, Rocky Mountain spotted fever, anthrax, tetanus, staph infections, strep throat, cholera, plague, meningococcal meningitis, gonorrhea, tuberculosis, leprosy, psittacosis (parrot fever), and trachoma.

VIRUSES

Structure   Most viruses are about 10 nanometers in diameter, about half the size of a ribosome. Many scientists do not consider viruses to be living cells, since they cannot reproduce themselves without the use of host cell nuclear structures and have no enzymes to synthesize ATP (energy) or to carry out other metabolic reactions. For this reason they are called *virions* (or virus particles). A virion has two basic structures: a *core*, which consists of nucleic acid (usually a single molecule of RNA or DNA); and a *capsid*, a protein coat that surrounds the nucleic acid and determines what type of cell to which the virus can attach itself. Other lipids, proteins, and glycoproteins are present in some viruses.

Classification   Viruses may be divided into two basic groups: DNA viruses and RNA viruses.

Diseases   Diseases caused by viruses include smallpox, cold sores (herpes simplex virus), polio, influenza, yellow fever, rabies, equine encephalitis, mumps, measles, and AIDS. Both DNA and RNA viruses may be oncogenic (cancer-producing). The genetic information of the infecting virus is incorporated into the DNA of the host cell, transforming it into a cancer (tumor) cell.

FUNGI   (singular : Fungus)

Fungi are plantlike organisms; examples are mushrooms, yeasts, molds, rusts, etc. They cannot be classified as plants because they contain no chlorophyll (inability to make their own food by photosynthesis). Diseases caused by fungi include vaginal yeast infection, "athlete's foot," thrush (infects mucous membranes), ringworm, diaper rash, and jock itch.

PROTOZOA   (singular : Protozoon)

Diseases caused by protozoa (one-celled animals) include malaria, amoebic dysentery, and African sleeping sickness.

PARASITIC WORMS

Parasitic worms that are hazardous to humans include lung flukes, liver flukes, blood flukes (cause schistosomiasis), tapeworms, hookworms, Trichinella (cause trichinosis), Ascaris, whipworms, and pinworms.

BACTERIA

The shapes of various bacteria as seen through a light microscope

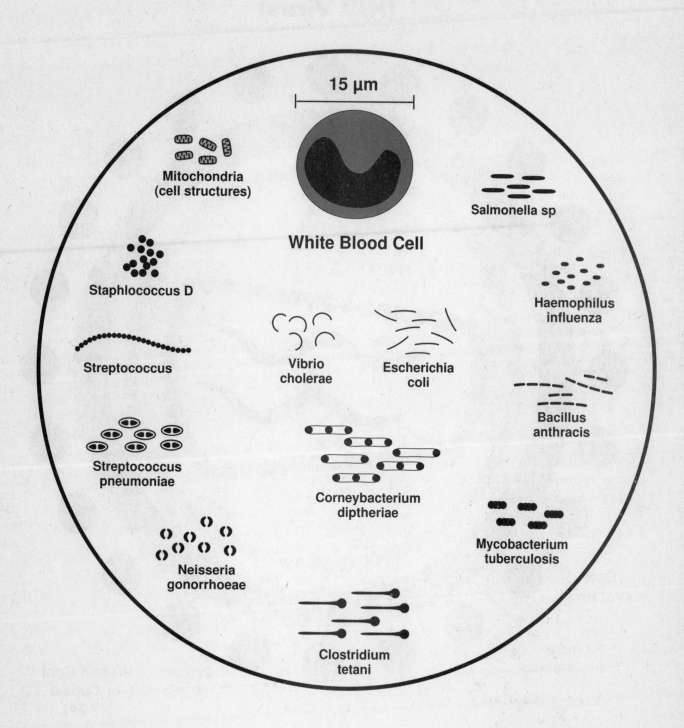

15 µm

Mitochondria
(cell structures)

White Blood Cell

Salmonella sp

Staphlococcus D

Haemophilus
influenza

Streptococcus

Vibrio
cholerae

Escherichia
coli

Bacillus
anthracis

Streptococcus
pneumoniae

Corneybacterium
diptheriae

Mycobacterium
tuberculosis

Neisseria
gonorrhoeae

Clostridium
tetani

VIRUSES

Human Immunodeficiency Virus
(HIV Virus)

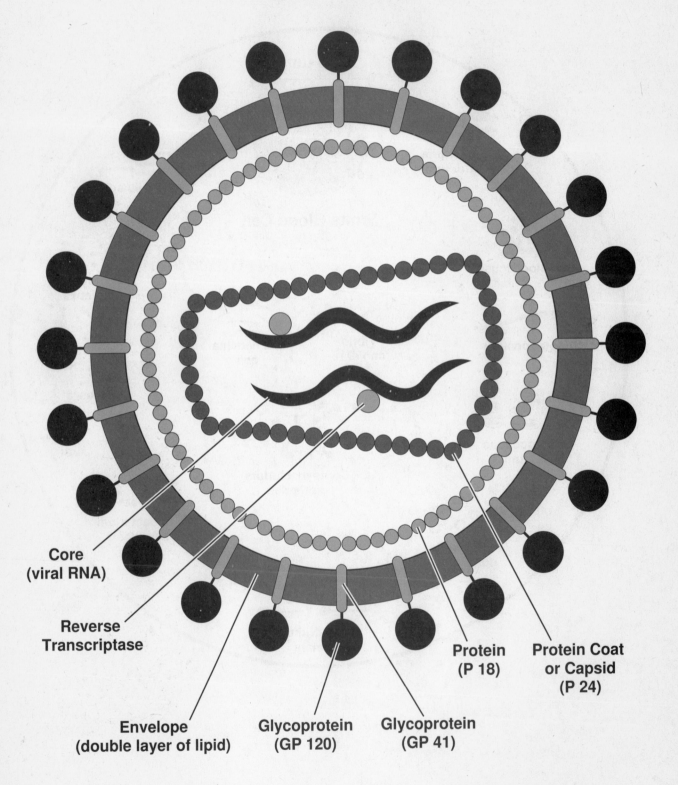

Core
(viral RNA)

Reverse
Transcriptase

Envelope
(double layer of lipid)

Glycoprotein
(GP 120)

Glycoprotein
(GP 41)

Protein
(P 18)

Protein Coat
or Capsid
(P 24)

PARASITES
Tapeworm (Taenia saginata)

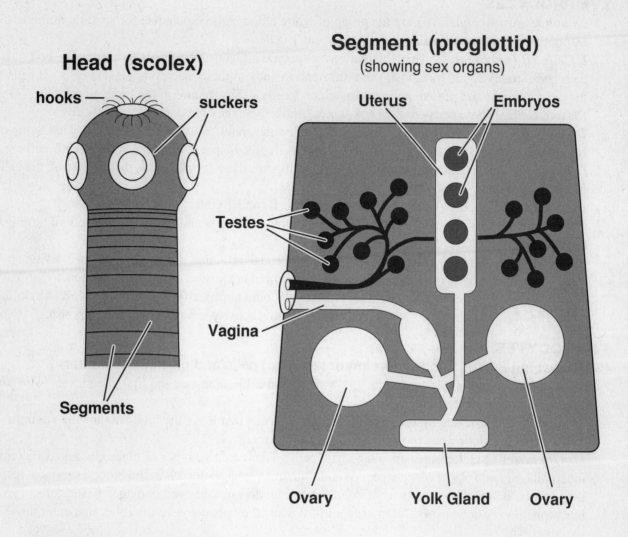

Head (scolex)

hooks —
suckers

Segments

Segment (proglottid)
(showing sex organs)

Uterus
Embryos
Testes
Vagina
Ovary
Yolk Gland
Ovary

Human Intestine

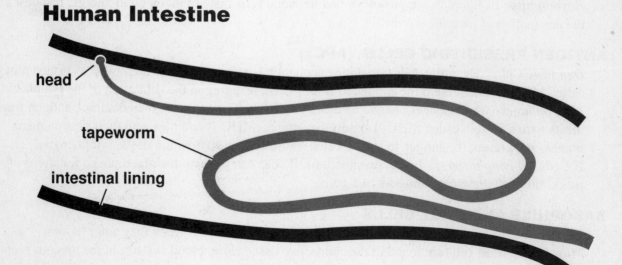

head
tapeworm
intestinal lining

INTRODUCTION / Effector Cells
(Cells Involved in Defense Mechanisms)

LYMPHOCYTES

Lymphocytes   Lymphocytes are the group of white blood cells responsible for specific immune responses; there are two main types: B cells and T cells.

B Cells (B lymphocytes)   Upon activation by specific antigens (chemicals foreign to the body), B cells proliferate (divide by mitosis) and differentiate into antibody-secreting plasma cells. B cells may also process and present antigens to helper T cells. They mature in the bone marrow.

Plasma Cells   These cells produce and secrete antibodies; they are derived from B cells.

T Cells (T lymphocytes)   The "T" refers to the thymus gland, where T cells mature. This group of lymphocytes includes three subclasses : cytotoxic T cells, helper T cells and suppressor T cells.

Cytotoxic T Cells   Upon activation by specific antigens, these lymphocytes directly attack the cell bearing that same type of antigen.

Helper T Cells   Helper T cells help to activate B cells and T cells.

Suppressor T Cells   Suppressor T cells inhibit cytotoxic T cells and antibody production, turning off an immune response.

Memory Cells   Memory cells include both B cells and T cells that have been produced during an initial infection; they respond rapidly during a subsequent exposure to the same antigen.

Natural Killer Cells (NK cells)   Natural killer cells bind nonspecifically to foreign cells and kill them directly. Since no prior exposure is required, this activity is not an immune response.

PHAGOCYTES
(Cells that ingest and destroy foreign or worn-out cells and particulate matter)

Neutrophils   Neutrophils are phagocytic white blood cells. They are the first phagocytes to arrive at a site of infection or tissue damage.

Monocytes   Monocytes are phagocytic white blood cells that leave the bloodstream and are transformed into wandering macrophages in the tissue spaces.

Macrophages   Macrophages are phagocytic cells. There are two types of macrophages: wandering macrophages and fixed macrophages. Wandering macrophages travel in the blood as monocytes; they exit blood capillaries in areas of infection and ingest microbes and damaged tissue cells. Fixed macrophages reside in many different types of tissues; they phagocytize microbes that enter these tissues.

Eosinophils   Eosinophils are phagocytic white blood cells that are involved in allergic responses and the destruction of parasitic worms.

ANTIGEN PRESENTING CELLS (APCs)

Dendritic Cells   Dendritic cells trap antigens on their surfaces, combine them with a surface protein called MHC-II, and present the antigen to B or T cells, resulting in the activation of the lymphocytes.

Macrophages   Macrophages phagocytize and partially digest antigens; then combine antigen fragments with a protein called MHC-II, insert the antigen–MHC-II complex into their plasma membranes, and present the antigen to B or T cells, resulting in the activation of the lymphocytes.

B Cells (B lymphocytes)   In certain situations, B cells can perform the macrophage functions of processing and presenting antigens to T cells.

BASOPHILS AND MAST CELLS

Basophils   Basophils are white blood cells that become mast cells when they enter tissues.

Mast Cells   Mast cells are found in the connective tissue along blood vessels, in the mucous membranes lining the gastrointestinal tract, and in the lungs. They secrete histamine, which causes local arterioles to dilate (increasing blood flow) and airways in the lungs to constrict (decreasing air flow).

8

TYPES OF EFFECTOR CELLS

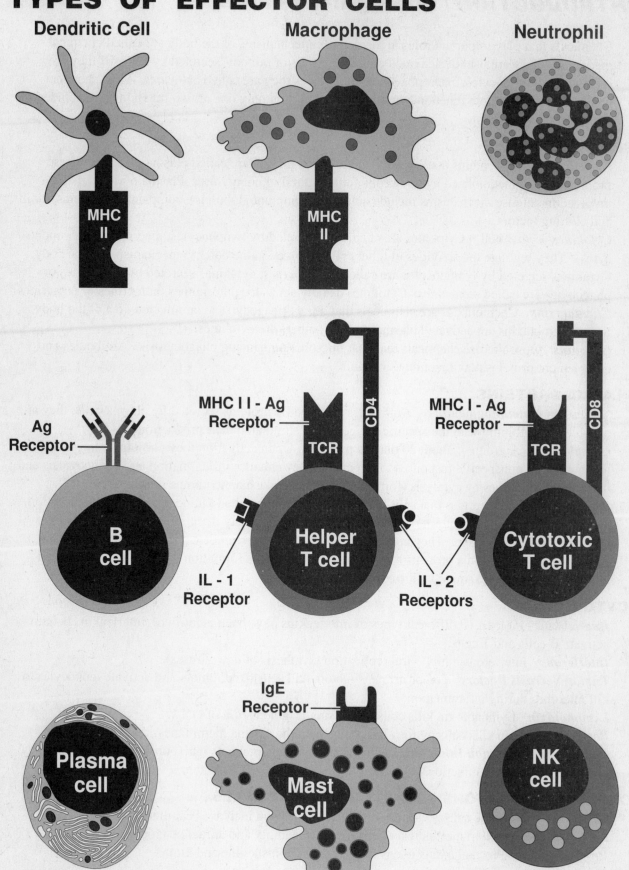

INTRODUCTION / Chemical Mediators

Chemicals that play important roles in the defense mechanisms of the body are called chemical mediators. They are usually activated plasma proteins or proteins secreted by cells. If they are secreted by lymphocytes, macrophages, or monocytes they are called *cytokines*. Most chemical mediators have multiple functions; in this brief discussion only one or two functions are included for each chemical mediator.

GENERAL TERMS

Plasma Proteins　Proteins that circulate in the blood plasma are called plasma proteins. These proteins are not metabolized by body cells for structural or energy uses. Plasma proteins that are involved in defense mechanisms include antibodies (immunoglobulins), complement proteins, kinins, and clotting factors.

Cytokines (*cyto* = cell)　Cytokines are chemicals secreted by lymphocytes, macrophages, or monocytes . They regulate the activities of other cells involved in the defense mechanisms of the body. Cytokines secreted by lymphocytes are called *lymphokines*; cytokines secreted by monocytes or phagocytes are called *monokines*. Cytokines usually act as local hormones (autocrines or paracrines).

Chemotaxins　Chemotaxins are chemicals that attract phagocytes to an infected area of the body. Some chemotaxins are activated plasma proteins, others are cytokines.

Opsonins　Opsonins are chemicals that coat microbes, enhancing phagocytosis. Antibodies and complement proteins may function as opsonins.

PLASMA PROTEINS

Antibodies (Immunoglobulins)　Antibodies are specific proteins secreted by plasma cells; they are capable of combining with the specific antigens that stimulated their production.

Complement　A group of about 20 plasma proteins. Upon activation they participate in specific (immune) and nonspecific responses to infection. They enhance inflammation and phagocytosis and directly kill microbes by cytolysis (forming holes in the plasma membrane of the microbe).

Kinins　Kinins are peptides that split from a plasma protein called kininogen during inflammation. They induce vasodilation of arterioles and increased permeability of capillaries near the site of infection or tissue damage. They also attract phagocytes and stimulate pain receptors.

Clotting Factors　Plasma proteins that mediate (regulate) the formation of blood clots are called clotting factors. An example is fibrinogen.

CYTOKINES

Interleukins　At least 10 different types of interleukins have been identified. Interleukins help to activate B cells and T cells.

Interferons　Interferons inhibit viral replication (synthesis of new viruses).

Tumor Necrosis Factors　Tumor necrosis factors kill sensitized tumors and activate leukocytes to kill microbes during inflammation.

Lymphotoxin　Lymphotoxin kills cells by causing fragmentation of DNA.

Perforin　Perforin kills cells by forming channels in the plasma membranes, causing cytolysis.

Macrophage Migration Inhibiting Factor　This cytokine prevents macrophages from migrating away from the site of infection.

CHEMICAL MEDIATORS SECRETED BY MAST CELLS

Histamine　Histamine causes vasodilation of arterioles and increased capillary permeability.

Leukotrienes　Leukotrienes increase capillary permeability and attract phagocytes.

Prostaglandins　Prostaglandins intensify the effects of histamine and kinins.

CHEMICAL MEDIATORS SECRETED BY DAMAGED CELLS

Histamine and prostaglandins are also secreted by damaged tissue cells.

MACROPHAGES

Microbes ingested by macrophages stimulate the release of tumor necrosis factor (TNF) and interleukin-1 (IL-1).

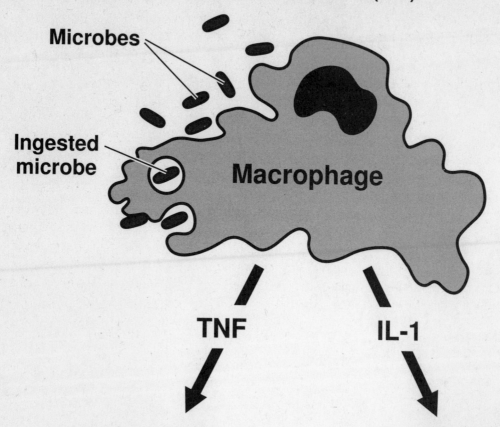

Microbes

Ingested microbe

Macrophage

TNF

IL-1

Leukocytes

stimulates accumulation at sites of inflammation

activates leukocytes to kill microbes

Macrophages

stimulates the synthesis of IL-1

Endothelial Cells and Fibroblasts

induces the synthesis of colony-stimulating factors

Body Cells

exerts an antiviral effect

Hypothalamus

induces fever

Lymphocytes

stimulates proliferation of B cells and T cells

Neutrophils

increases number of circulating neutrophils

Liver

stimulates production of immune substances

Hypothalamus

induces fever

2 Nonspecific Resistance

NONSPECIFIC RESISTANCE / The First Lines of Defense

The body's first lines of defense against infection are the barriers offered by surfaces exposed to the external environment: the skin and the mucous membranes.

SKIN

Basic Structure   The skin covers the body and protects underlying tissues from invasion by microbes; very few microbes can penetrate the intact skin. It has two principal parts: the epidermis and the dermis. The epidermis (outer layer) is composed of epithelial cells arranged in five layers.   The dermis (inner layer) is composed of connective tissue containing mast cells, fibroblasts, macrophages, and adipose cells enmeshed in collagen and elastic fibers.

Stratum Corneum   The outermost layer of the epidermis, called the stratum corneum, consists of flat, dead cells completely filled with a protein called keratin. These cells form a physical barrier that protects the deeper tissues from microbial invasion, abrasion, and dehydration.

Glandular Secretions   Perspiration, secreted by sudoriferous (sweat) glands, contains an enzyme called lysozyme, which breaks down the cell walls of certain bacteria. Lysozyme is also found in tears, saliva, nasal secretions, and tissue fluids. Sebum, secreted by sebaceous (oil) glands, contains unsaturated fatty acids which inhibit the growth of certain bacteria and fungi.

Harmless Bacteria   Harmless bacteria (called commensal bacteria) live on the skin. The presence of these bacteria suppresses the growth of other potentially more virulent types.

MUCOUS MEMBRANES

Mucous membranes protect the underlying tissues from microbes, but if present in sufficient numbers, certain microbes may be able to penetrate into the underlying connective tissues.

Basic Structure   The tracts of the body (gastrointestinal, respiratory, urinary, and reproductive tracts) are lined with mucous membranes. These mucous membranes have the same basic arrangement of tissues as the skin : an outer epithelial layer and an inner connective tissue layer.

Mucus   Specialized epithelial cells secrete a sticky fluid called mucus, which covers the surface of the mucous membranes and traps microbes and foreign substances. Some particles trapped by the mucus are phagocytized by macrophages that are present in the nearby lymphatic tissues.

Hairs   The mucous membranes of the nose contain mucus-coated hairs, which help to filter the incoming air. In this way the lungs are kept relatively free of microbes, dust, and pollutants.

Cilia   Many of the epithelial cells lining the upper respiratory tract have cilia (hairlike projections) that sweep back and forth, propelling the mucus toward the mouth, where it is swallowed.

Acid   Hydrochloric acid is secreted by cells in the lining of the stomach to aid in digestion. This strong acid (pH about 2.0) destroys many bacteria and bacterial toxins. Lactic acid is produced in the vagina by commensal bacteria that metabolize the glycogen secreted by epithelial cells; the resulting acidic environment inhibits invasion by pathogens.

Flushing   Infections in the kidney tubules, bladder and urethra are minimized by the constant production and flow of urine. Microbes are continously flushed from the system.

Harmless (Commensal) Bacteria   Harmless bacteria live in the large intestines. The presence of these bacteria suppress the growth of other potentially more virulent types.

Tears   A thin, transparent mucous membrane called the *conjunctiva* covers the anterior portion of the eye up to the cornea and the internal surface of the eyelids. The corneas of the eyes consist of living cells that are in direct contact with the external environment. Tears, produced by the lacrimal apparatus, protect the conjunctiva and cornea from bacterial infection; they contain the enzyme *lysozyme* which digests bacterial cell walls, killing the bacteria.

NONSPECIFIC BARRIERS TO INFECTION

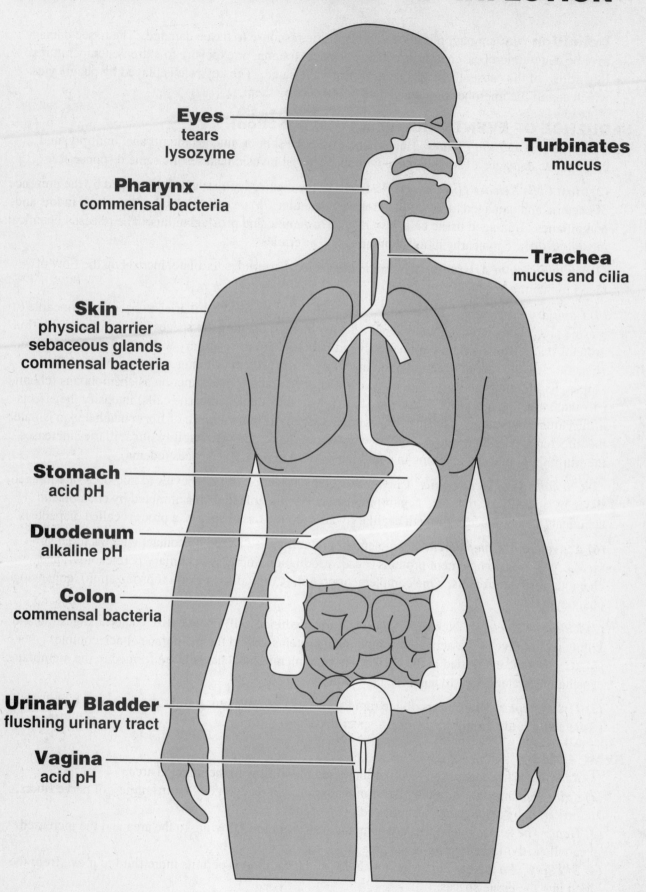

Eyes
tears
lysozyme

Turbinates
mucus

Pharynx
commensal bacteria

Trachea
mucus and cilia

Skin
physical barrier
sebaceous glands
commensal bacteria

Stomach
acid pH

Duodenum
alkaline pH

Colon
commensal bacteria

Urinary Bladder
flushing urinary tract

Vagina
acid pH

NONSPECIFIC RESISTANCE / Inflammation

Definition   Inflammation is a local, nonspecific response to tissue damage. The tissue damage may be due to microbes, chemical irritants, physical trauma, or exposure to extreme temperatures. Regardless of the cause, the response is basically the same. The key role is played by phagocytes, which engulf the microbes or damaged cells and destroy them.

SEQUENCE OF EVENTS (for a bacterial infection)

(1) Bacteria Enter the Tissues   Bacteria penetrate the skin or mucous membrane, multiply, and cause tissue damage. (Tissue damage without bacterial invasion causes the same response.)

(2) Mast Cells Release Histamine   Mast cells in the connective tissue are stimulated by the presence of bacteria and damaged tissue cells to release histamine. Mast cells also release prostaglandins and leukotrienes. Damaged tissue cells also release histamine and prostaglandins. The released chemical mediators diffuse to nearby blood capillaries and arterioles.

(3) Vasodilation of Arterioles   Histamine causes local arterioles to dilate, increasing the flow of blood to the infected area.

(4) Capillary Permeability Is Increased   Histamine causes local capillaries to become permeable to plasma proteins by inducing endothelial cells to contract, opening the spaces between them. Plasma proteins that mediate inflammation are able to pass through the capillary wall into the infected area. Histamine triggers the conversion of an inactive plasma protein (kininogen) into peptides called kinins. Kinins enhance vasodilation and capillary permeability and function as chemotaxins (chemicals that attract phagocytes). Prostaglandins (released by damaged tissue cells) intensify the effects of histamine and kinins. Clotting factors are activated, forming a mesh of fibrin that helps to isolate the infected area and prevent the spread of bacteria. Increased permeability of capillaries increases the filtration of plasma, resulting in a buildup of fluid in the tissue spaces (edema).

(5) Chemotaxis of Neutrophils   Chemotaxis is the attraction of phagocytes to microbes or damaged tissue by a chemical stimulus. Neutrophils migrate to the infected area attracted by chemotactic chemicals. They squeeze through capillary walls into the tissue spaces, a process called diapedesis.

(6) Activation of Complement   Complement proteins are activated by contact with bacterial surfaces. Activated complement proteins cause vasodilation, increased capillary permeability, and chemotaxis of neutrophils. One complement protein (C3b) coats bacteria (opsonization), enhancing phagocytosis.

(7) Killing of Bacteria   Neutrophils (a type of white blood cell) phagocytize bacteria, digesting and killing them. Five of the activated complement proteins, called the membrane attack complex (MAC), become embedded in the bacterial plasma membrane; channels are formed in the membrane, causing the bacterial cell to burst (lysis) and die.

(8) Tissue Repair   Fibroblasts divide rapidly and secrete collagen, forming scar tissue. Usually local tissue cells divide, forming new organ-specific cells.

SYMPTOMS

(1) Redness   The redness is a result of increased blood flow to the infected area.
(2) Pain   Pain may be caused by the stimulation of pain receptors by kinins, injury of nerve fibers, and irritation by toxic chemicals released by microbes.
(3) Heat   The heat is due to the large amount of warm blood flowing to the area and the increased metabolic activities occurring in the area.
(4) Swelling   An increase in the permeability of the capillaries permits more fluid to move from the blood into the tissue spaces.

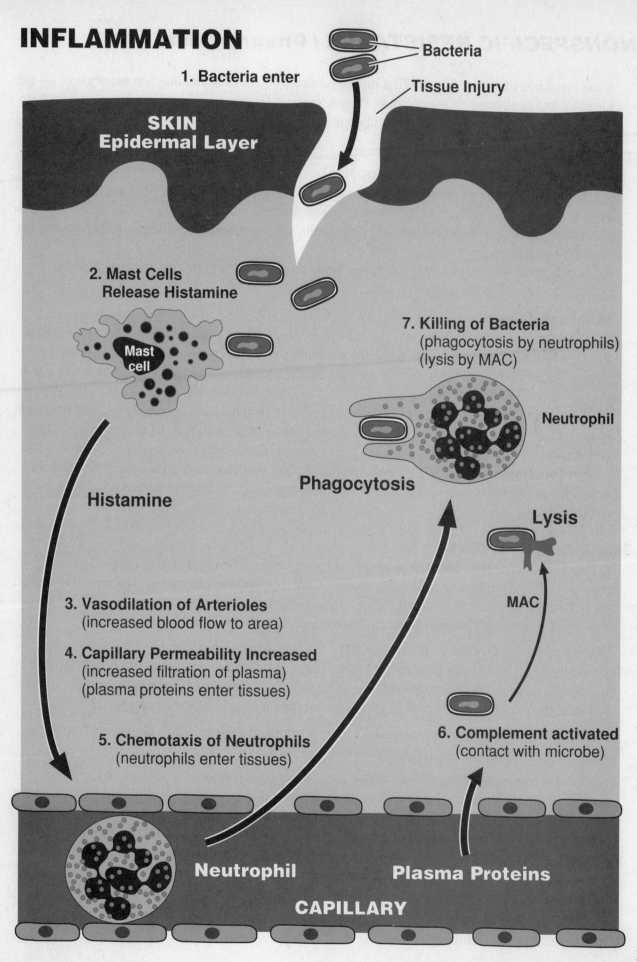

INFLAMMATION

Bacteria

1. Bacteria enter

Tissue Injury

SKIN
Epidermal Layer

2. Mast Cells
Release Histamine

Mast cell

7. Killing of Bacteria
(phagocytosis by neutrophils)
(lysis by MAC)

Neutrophil

Phagocytosis

Histamine

Lysis

MAC

3. Vasodilation of Arterioles
(increased blood flow to area)

4. Capillary Permeability Increased
(increased filtration of plasma)
(plasma proteins enter tissues)

5. Chemotaxis of Neutrophils
(neutrophils enter tissues)

6. Complement activated
(contact with microbe)

Neutrophil

Plasma Proteins

CAPILLARY

17

NONSPECIFIC RESISTANCE / Phagocytosis

Most microbes that penetrate the first lines of defense — the skin and mucous membranes — are ingested and destroyed by phagocytes. Phagocytosis is the process by which phagocytes ingest and destroy microbes or foreign particulate matter.

TYPES OF PHAGOCYTES
Granulocytes   (Granular Leukocytes)
(1) Neutrophils   The most actively phagocytic type of white blood cell. They are the first phagocytes to arrive at a site of infection or tissue damage.

(2) Eosinophils   Eosinophils are white blood cells that are involved in allergic responses and the destruction of parasitic worms.

(3) Monocytes   Monocytes are phagocytic white blood cells that migrate to infected areas, enlarge, and develop into wandering macrophages.

Macrophages
(1) Wandering Macrophages   Wandering macrophages travel (wander) throughout the body in the blood plasma as monocytes. They are attracted to damaged tissue areas by chemotaxis during inflammation. When the monocytes leave the blood and enter infected tissues they grow into larger cells called macrophages.

(2) Fixed Macrophages   Fixed macrophages reside in lymph nodes, spleen and other tissues and organs. The following list includes locations and names of the major fixed macrophages: skin (histiocytes); bone marrow (macrophage precursors); lymph nodes (macrophages); spleen (splenic macrophages); brain (microglia); liver (stellate reticuloendothelial cells or Kupffer cells); lungs (alveolar macrophages); kidneys (mesangial macrophages); synovial joints (synovial A cells).

SEQUENCE OF EVENTS
(1) Adherence (contact between microbe and phagocyte)   The first step in phagocytosis is contact and binding between the surfaces of the microbe and the phagocyte. Bacteria surrounded by polysaccharide capsules resist binding. In order to establish firm contact (adherence), they first must be coated (opsonized) by antibodies or certain complement fragments (C3b).

(2) Ingestion (endocytosis)   If adherence is adequate, it triggers ingestion of the microbe by endocytosis. Pseudopodia (temporary extensions of the plasma membrane) projected from the phagocyte surround the microbe and fuse. The portion of the plasma membrane surrounding the microbe pinches off and enters the cytoplasm, forming a vesicle called a phagosome.

(3) Phagosome (fusion with a lysosome)   The phagosome merges with a lysosome, forming a single, larger vesicle called a phagolysosome.

(4) Phagolysosome (killing of microbe)   Inside the phagolysosome most bacteria are killed within 10 to 30 minutes. The phagolysosome has several mechanisms for killing. It contains the enzyme lysozyme, which breaks down bacterial cell walls; it also contains digestive (hydrolytic) enzymes that degrade carbohydrates, lipids, proteins, and nucleic acids. Enzymes in the phagolysome membrane produce hydrogen peroxide and other lethal oxygen derivatives that are extremely destructive to macromolecules in a process called the *respiratory (oxidative) burst.*

(5) Exocytosis Substances that cannot be further degraded remain in structures called *residual bodies*. Residual bodies migrate to the plasma membrane, fuse with it, and release their contents into the extracellular fluid by exocytosis.

PHAGOCYTOSIS
Neutrophils and macrophages phagocytize bacteria, virus-infected cells, cancer cells, and foreign materials

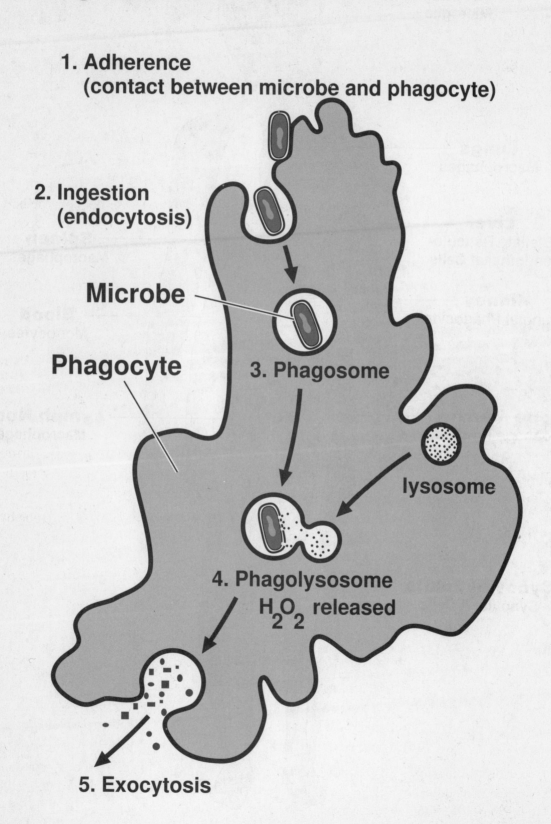

1. Adherence
(contact between microbe and phagocyte)

2. Ingestion
(endocytosis)

Microbe

Phagocyte

3. Phagosome

lysosome

4. Phagolysosome
H_2O_2 released

5. Exocytosis

MACROPHAGE LOCATIONS

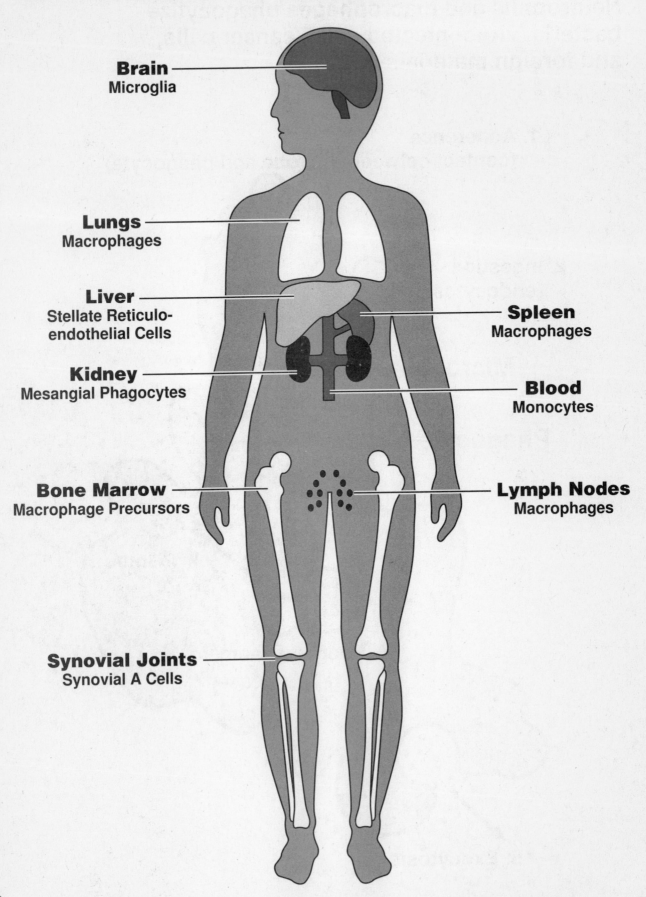

Brain
Microglia

Lungs
Macrophages

Liver
Stellate Reticulo-
endothelial Cells

Kidney
Mesangial Phagocytes

Bone Marrow
Macrophage Precursors

Synovial Joints
Synovial A Cells

Spleen
Macrophages

Blood
Monocytes

Lymph Nodes
Macrophages

ALVEOLAR MACROPHAGES
Location of macrophages in the air sacs (alveoli) of the lungs

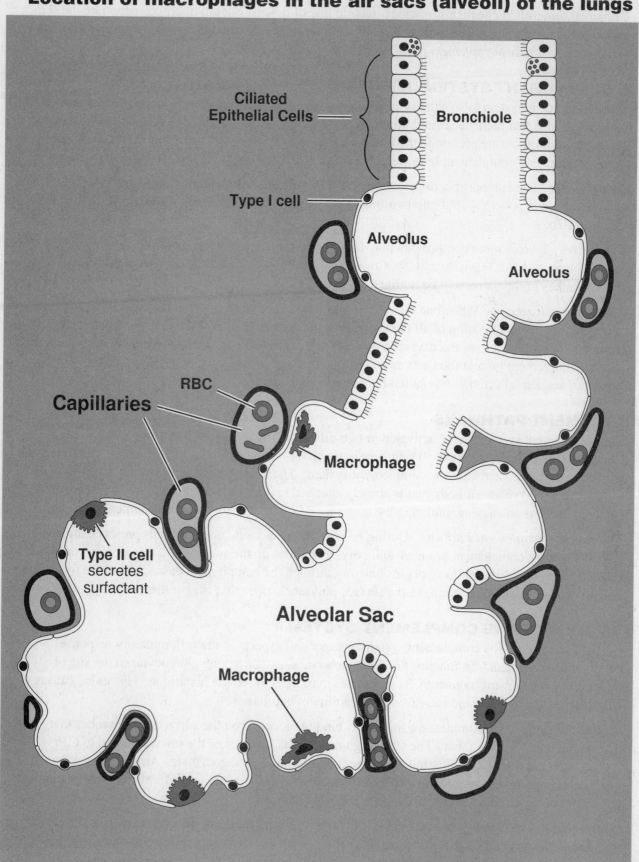

Ciliated Epithelial Cells

Bronchiole

Type I cell

Alveolus

Alveolus

RBC

Capillaries

Macrophage

Type II cell secretes surfactant

Alveolar Sac

Macrophage

NONSPECIFIC RESISTANCE / Complement System

Certain antimicrobial chemicals provide a second line of defense should microbes penetrate the skin and mucous membranes. The most important antimicrobial substances activated or released during inflammation are the *complement proteins* and *interferons*.

THE COMPLEMENT SYSTEM DEFINED

The complement system (also called complement proteins or complement) is a complex system of plasma proteins that mediate several important defense mechanisms. Prior to activation, most of the complement proteins are present in the blood plasma as enzyme precursors (proenzymes). These proteins are called complement because they "complement" or enhance the inflammatory response.

Components The components of the complement system are designated by numbers: C1, C2, C3, etc. When a component is split into two fragments, letters are added: C2 is split (cleaved), forming C2a and C2b.

Complexes Two or more components may bind to form a complex. For example, the membrane attack complex (MAC) consists of C5b, C6, C7, C8, and C9. In this discussion the functions of a few of the key components will be outlined.

Complement Cascade When one complement protein is activated, it triggers a chain reaction, which results in the activation of all the proteins in the complement system. The first activated complement protein acts as an enzyme that causes the activation of a second complement protein; the second complement protein then acts as an enzyme that activates a third protein, and so on. This system of sequential activation is called the complement cascade.

COMPLEMENT PATHWAYS

The complement system can be activated in two different ways.

Classical Complement Pathway During an immune (specific) response, the formation of antigen-antibody complexes activates the complement system. The complement fragment C1 binds to the stem (Fc portion) of an antibody that is already attached to it specific antigen. The C1 is then activated and acts as an enzyme, initiating the sequence of reactions called the complement cascade.

Alternative Complement Pathway During nonspecific responses (no antibodies present), direct contact between complement proteins and polysaccharides on the surface of a microbe activates the system. The alternative pathway begins halfway through the complement cascade with the formation of C3b. Only certain microbes have the surface polysaccharides that trigger this pathway.

FUNCTIONS OF THE COMPLEMENT SYSTEM

(1) Inflammation The complement system enhances all aspects of the inflammatory response. Complement fragment C5a functions as a chemotactic agent, attracting phagocytes to the site of infection. Complement fragment C3a stimulates mast cells to release histamine. Histamine causes vasodilation of arterioles and increased permeability of capillaries.

(2) Phagocytosis C3b complement fragments bind to receptors on the surfaces of microbes that resist adherence, coating them. The C3b fragments on the surfaces of the microbes bind to C3b receptors on phagocytes, facilitating adherence and promoting phagocytosis. Any substance that binds to foreign molecules and induces their phagocytosis is called an *opsonin*; the process of coating a foreign cell or particle with opsonins is called *opsonization*.

(3) Cytolysis The membrane attack complex (MAC) punches holes in the plasma membrane of a microbe. This process, called cytolysis (also called *lysis*), causes the membrane to rupture, killing the microbe.

COMPLEMENT SYSTEM
Alternative Complement Pathway (nonspecific response)

Microbes
contact between complement proteins
and
polysaccharides on surface of microbe
activate complement

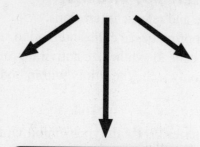

Phagocytosis
C3b
enhances phagocytosis
by opsonization
of microbes

Inflammation
C3a
stimulates mast cells
to release histamine

C5a
activates phagocytes
and attracts them to site

Cytolysis
MAC
penetrates microbe
plasma membrane,
causing lysis

Phagocytosis
Opsonization of microbe enhances phagocytosis

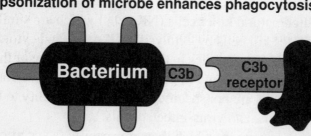

Bacterium | C3b | C3b receptor | Macrophage

Cytolysis
MAC (membrane attack complex)
C5b, C6, C7, C8, C9 penetrate the plasma
membrane, lysing and killing the cell

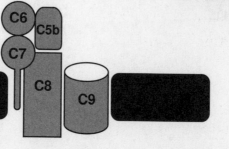

Plasma Membrane of Microbe

NONSPECIFIC RESISTANCE / Interferons and NK Cells

INTERFERONS (IFNs)

Interferons are proteins produced by certain types of body cells infected with viruses. Cells capable of producing interferons include macrophages, helper T cells, cytotoxic T cells, NK cells, and fibroblasts. Interferons inhibit viral replication. The action of interferons is nonspecific — that is, they act against a large number of different viruses.

Mechanism for Suppression of Viruses

(1) Virus-infected cells produce and release interferons.
(2) Interferons diffuse to neighboring tissue cells and bind to surface receptors.
(3) Interferons stimulate tissue cells to synthesize antiviral proteins that inhibit viral replication. (Viruses can cause disease only if they multiply within body cells.)

Types of Interferons

There are two main types of interferons (both types inhibit viral replication):

(1) Type I Interferons Type I interferons include alpha-interferon and beta-interferon. Type I interferons suppress the formation of certain types of tumors and inhibit tumor metastases (spreading of cancer cells to other parts of the body). Alpha-interferon is approved in the United States for the treatment of virus-associated disorders, such as Kaposi's sarcoma, a cancer that often occurs in patients with AIDS. It is also used to treat genital warts (caused by the herpes virus) and hepatitis C (caused by the hepatitis C virus).

(2) Type II Interferon Type II interferon is also called gamma-interferon. NK cells and cytotoxic T cells secrete gamma-interferon, which activates neutrophils and macrophages, greatly increasing their phagocytic activity. Gamma-interferon secreted by NK cells also acts as an autocrine, enhancing the cell-killing activities of the cells that secreted it.

NATURAL KILLER CELLS (NK Cells)

There is a population of lymphocytes called natural killer cells (NK cells) which are similar to cytotoxic T cells. Both types of lymphocytes kill cells by cytolysis. NK cells (and cytotoxic T cells) secrete a cytokine called *perforin*, which forms holes in the plasma membrane of the target cell, causing it to burst and die. NK cells are found in the lymph nodes, spleen, bone marrow, and blood. The actions of the NK cells are nonspecific; they have the ability to kill a wide variety of infectious microbes, tumor cells, and virus-infected cells.

Cytotoxic T cells attack cells that bear antigens for which they are specific (a specific or immune response), while NK cells attack cells without interacting with antigens or other lymphocytes (a nonspecific response). NK cells also produce interferon, which inhibits viral replication. NK cells are defective or decreased in number in some cancer patients and in patients with AIDS.

INTERFERONS AND NK CELLS

Interferons nonspecifically block viral replication.

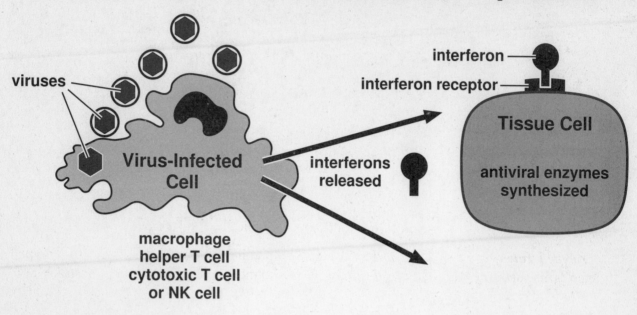

viruses

Virus-Infected
Cell

macrophage
helper T cell
cytotoxic T cell
or NK cell

interferons
released

interferon

interferon receptor

Tissue Cell

antiviral enzymes
synthesized

NK cells nonspecifically kill cancer cells.

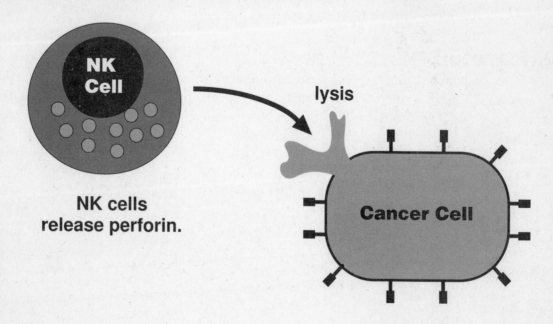

**NK
Cell**

NK cells
release perforin.

lysis

Cancer Cell

3 Lymphatic Tissues

LYMPHATIC TISSUES / Overview

LYMPHATIC TISSUE

Reticular Connective Tissue Lymphatic tissue is a specialized form of reticular connective tissue. It consists of reticular cells and reticular fibers that form a 3-dimensional mesh. Large numbers of lymphocytes (B cells and T cells), phagocytes (macrophages), and dendritic cells (antigen-presenting cells) occupy the spaces in the mesh.

Stem Cells All lymphocytes are derived from undifferentiated stem cells in the bone marrow. The stem cells differentiate into millions of different T cells and B cells, each programmed to respond to a particular antigen.

B Cells When stimulated by the appropriate antigen, a B cell divides and differentiates, producing a clone (population of genetically identical cells) of antibody-secreting plasma cells and memory B cells. B cells are responsible for antibody-mediated immune responses.

T Cells When a T cell is stimulated by the appropriate antigen a similar response occurs: it divides and differentiates, producing a clone of activated T cells and memory T cells. T cells are responsible for cell-mediated immune responses.

LYMPH AND LYMPHATIC VESSELS

About three liters of excess interstitial fluid is produced daily by the filtration of blood plasma. This excess fluid is drained from the tissue spaces by lymphatic vessels and returned to the blood. Closed-ended lymphatic capillaries converge into larger tubes called lymphatic vessels, which empty into still larger lymph trunks. The lymph trunks merge, forming lymphatic ducts that empty into the right and left subclavian veins. Although the fluid inside lymphatic vessels is identical to interstitial fluid, it is called lymph.

PRIMARY LYMPHATIC ORGANS

The primary lymphatic organs (bone marrow and thymus gland) are the locations where lymphocytes mature. When they mature they are said to be *immunocompetent* (capable of carrying out immune responses).

Bone Marrow B cells mature in the bone marrow. Mature B cells migrate via the blood to secondary lymphatic organs and tissues.

Thymus Gland T cells mature in the thymus. Immature T cells migrate from the bone marrow to the thymus gland, which is located in the thorax anterior to the heart and major blood vessels. Mature T cells migrate via the blood from the thymus to secondary lymphatic organs and tissues.

SECONDARY LYMPHATIC ORGANS

B and T cells reside in the secondary lymphatic organs (lymph nodes and spleen) and interact with antigens in the blood and lymph. Most immune responses occur in the secondary lymphatic organs.

Lymph Nodes Lymph nodes are found throughout the body along the course of lymphatic vessels. They filter the lymph.

Spleen The spleen is located in the upper left of the abdomen behind the stomach and just below the diaphragm. It filters the blood.

DIFFUSE LYMPHATIC TISSUE

Lymphatic Nodules   When lymphatic tissue is not enclosed by a capsule, it is called diffuse or unencapsulated lymphatic tissue. It consists of lymphatic nodules (follicles) embedded in reticular connective tissue. Lymphatic nodules are found in almost every organ of the body, especially in the mucous membranes lining the tracts (gastrointestinal, respiratory, urinary, and reproductive). Most nodules are solitary structures scattered in the lamina propria (connective tissue layer) of mucous membranes. Other nodules occur in multiple, large aggregations; examples include the tonsils, Peyer's patches of the ileum, and the vermiform appendix. Diffuse lymphatic tissue contains B cells.

LYMPHATIC SYSTEM

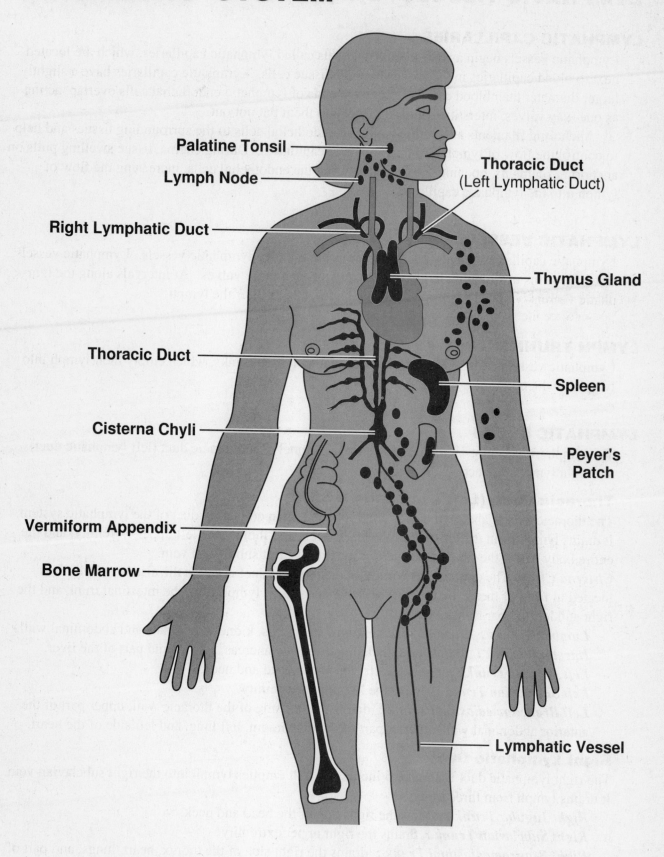

Palatine Tonsil

Lymph Node

Right Lymphatic Duct

Thoracic Duct

Cisterna Chyli

Vermiform Appendix

Bone Marrow

Thoracic Duct
(Left Lymphatic Duct)

Thymus Gland

Spleen

Peyer's
Patch

Lymphatic Vessel

LYMPHATIC TISSUES / Lymphatic Vessels

LYMPHATIC CAPILLARIES

Lymphatic vessels begin as closed-ended vessels called lymphatic capillaries, which are located next to blood capillaries in the spaces between tissue cells. Lymphatic capillaries have a slightly larger diameter than blood capillaries and the ends of lymphatic endothelial cells overlap, acting as one-way valves; interstitial fluid can flow into them but not out.

Anchoring filaments attach the lymphatic endothelial cells to the surrounding tissues and help to control the flow of lymph into the lymphatic capillaries. During edema, tissue swelling pulls on anchoring filaments, opening the spaces between the endothelial cells, increasing the flow of lymph into the lymphatic capillaries.

LYMPHATIC VESSELS

Lymphatic capillaries converge to form larger tubes called lymphatic vessels. Lymphatic vessels resemble veins in structure, but have thinner walls and more valves. At intervals along the lymphatic vessels lymph flows through lymph nodes, which filter the lymph.

LYMPH TRUNKS

Lymphatic vessels unite to form larger tubes called lymph trunks, which empty their lymph into lymphatic ducts.

LYMPHATIC DUCTS

The lymph trunks empty lymph into two main channels: the thoracic duct (left lymphatic duct) and right lymphatic duct.

Thoracic Duct (Left Lymphatic Duct)

The thoracic duct is about 16 inches long. It is the main collecting duct of the lymphatic system. It drains lymph from the left side of the head, neck, and thorax, the left upper extremity, and the entire body below the ribs. It empties lymph into the left subclavian vein.

Cisterna Chyli   The dilated first portion of the thoracic duct is called the cisterna chyli. It is located in front of the second lumbar vertebra and drains lymph from the intestinal trunk and the right and left lumbar trunks.

Lumbar Trunks : drain the lower extremities, pelvis, kidneys, adrenals and abdominal wall.

Intestinal Trunk : drains the stomach, intestines, pancreas, spleen, and part of the liver.

Left Jugular Trunk : drains the left side of the head and neck.

Left Subclavian Trunk : drains the left upper extremity.

Left Bronchomediastinal Trunk : drains the left side of the thoracic wall, upper part of the anterior abdominal wall, anterior part of the diaphragm, left lung, and left side of the heart.

Right Lymphatic Duct

The right lymphatic duct is about 0.5 inches long. It empties lymph into the right subclavian vein. It drains lymph from three trunks.

Right Jugular Trunk : drains the right side of the head and neck.

Right Subclavian Trunk : drains the right upper extremity.

Right Broncomediastinal Trunk : drains the right side of the thorax, heart, lungs, and part of the liver.

LYMPHATIC VESSELS

Lymphatic Vessels

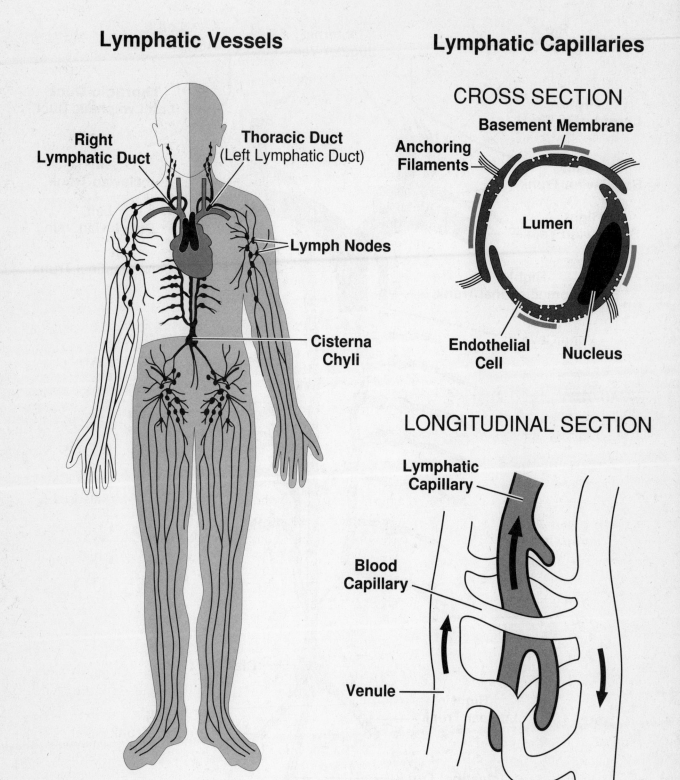

Right Lymphatic Duct

Thoracic Duct
(Left Lymphatic Duct)

Lymph Nodes

Cisterna Chyli

Lymphatic Capillaries

CROSS SECTION

Basement Membrane

Anchoring Filaments

Lumen

Endothelial Cell

Nucleus

LONGITUDINAL SECTION

Lymphatic Capillary

Blood Capillary

Venule

Arteriole

LYMPH TRUNKS AND LYMPHATIC DUCTS

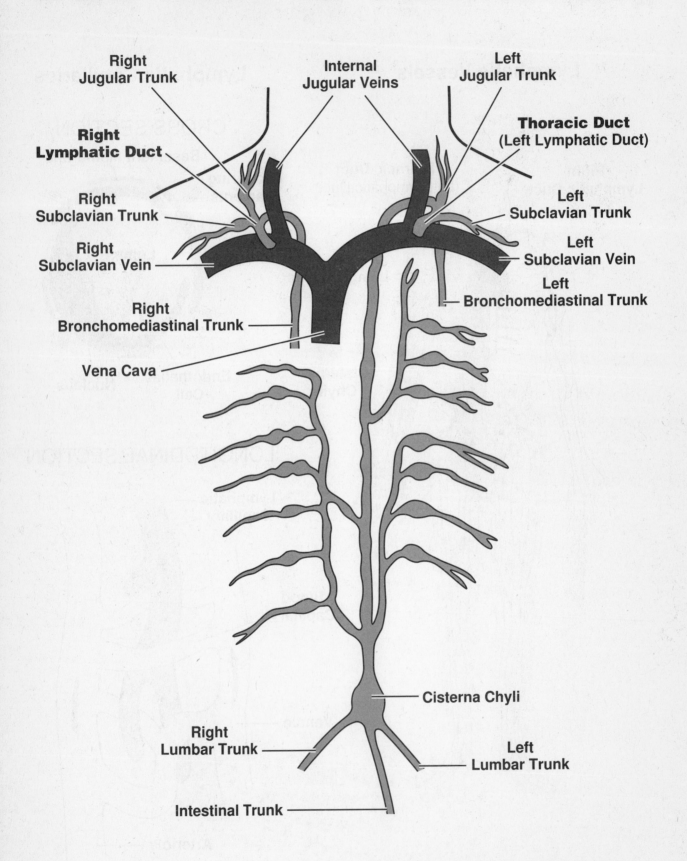

Right Jugular Trunk

Internal Jugular Veins

Left Jugular Trunk

Right Lymphatic Duct

Thoracic Duct (Left Lymphatic Duct)

Right Subclavian Trunk

Left Subclavian Trunk

Right Subclavian Vein

Left Subclavian Vein

Right Bronchomediastinal Trunk

Left Bronchomediastinal Trunk

Vena Cava

Cisterna Chyli

Right Lumbar Trunk

Left Lumbar Trunk

Intestinal Trunk

LYMPH AND BLOOD FLOW
The relationship between the lymphatic and cardiovascular systems

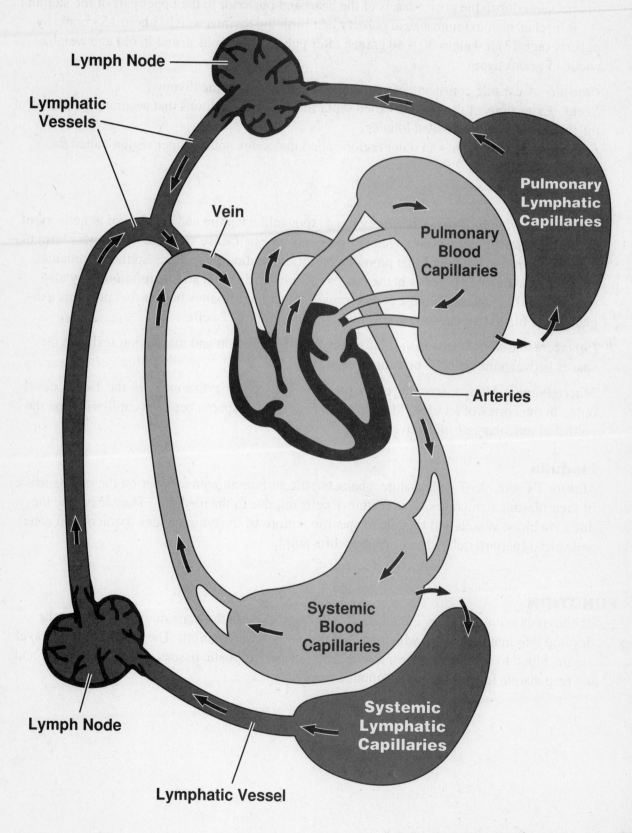

Lymph Node

Lymphatic Vessels

Vein

Pulmonary Lymphatic Capillaries

Pulmonary Blood Capillaries

Arteries

Systemic Blood Capillaries

Systemic Lymphatic Capillaries

Lymph Node

Lymphatic Vessel

LYMPHATIC TISSUES / Thymus Gland

STRUCTURE

The thymus is a soft structure consisting of two lobes (bilobed). It is located in the chest (thorax) anterior to the great vessels of the heart and posterior to the upper part of the sternum.

It reaches its maximum size at puberty. At birth the thymus weighs about 15 grams; by puberty (age 13) it weighs 30 – 40 grams; after puberty it atrophies, and in old age weighs about 15 grams again.

Capsule A capsule consisting of connective tissue envelops the thymus.
Septa Extensions of the capsule called septa form partial partitions that separate the tissues of the thymus into regions called lobules.
Lobules Each lobule has an outer region called the cortex and an inner region called the medulla.

Cortex

Epithelial Reticular Cells The cortex has a spongelike texture and consists of a network of epithelial reticular cells bound together by desmosomes. Dense granules in the cytoplasm of these cells secrete hormones that promote the differentiation of T cells. Epithelial reticular cells envelop groups of T cells in the process of mitotic division and maturation; they also surround all blood vessels in the cortex, providing a blood-thymus barrier that prevents antigens in the blood from making contact with the developing T cells.

Immature T Cells T cells in various stages of differentiation and maturation reside in the spaces between the reticular cells of the cortex.

Macrophages Many macrophages are present. They phagocytize many of the T cells developing in the cortex of lobules. Macrophages reside in the spaces between capillaries and the epithelial reticular cells that cover the capillaries.

Medulla

Mature T Cells As T cells mature, characteristic surface antigens appear on the outer surfaces of their plasma membranes. The mature T cells migrate to the medulla. They leave the medulla via blood vessels and migrate to specific regions of the lymph nodes (paracortical zone) and spleen (periarteriolar sheaths of the white pulp).

FUNCTION

The thymus is colonized by immature T cells originating in the bone marrow. These cells develop into mature T cells, which are released into the circulation. The mature T cells travel via the blood to the lymph nodes, spleen, and diffuse lymphatic tissues, where they reside and are responsible for cell-mediated immune responses.

THYMUS GLAND

Immature T Cells : Immature T cells migrate from the bone marrow via the blood to the thymus, where they mature.

Mature T Cells : Mature T cells migrate from the thymus to specific regions in the lymph nodes and the spleen, where they reside.

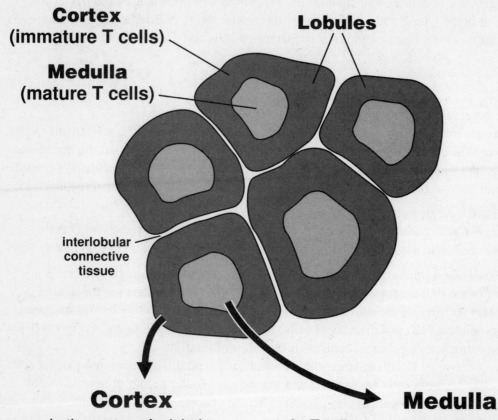

Cortex
(immature T cells)

Medulla
(mature T cells)

Lobules

interlobular connective tissue

Cortex

In the cortex of a lobule, reticular cells envelop groups of T cells that are multiplying and maturing.

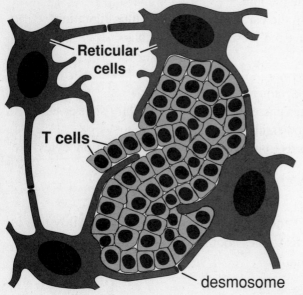

Reticular cells

T cells

desmosome

Medulla

As T cells mature, they migrate to the medulla. Fully mature T cells leave the medulla via venules and efferent lymphatic vessels.

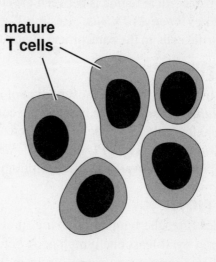

mature T cells

LYMPHATIC TISSUES / Lymph Nodes

STRUCTURE

Lymph nodes are spherical or kidney-shaped. A depression called the *hilus* (or hilum), where arteries and nerves enter and veins exit, is located on the concave side. Lymph nodes are found throughout the body along the course of lymphatic vessels. They are abundant under the arms, in the groin area, along the great vessels of the neck, and in the thorax and abdomen. Lymph nodes are covered by a *capsule* of dense connective tissue; extensions of the capsule called *trabeculae* form partitions within the lymph nodes. A network of reticular fibers ensheathed by *reticular cells* extends throughout the node; mature (immunocompetent) B cells and T cells are suspended throughout.

CORTEX

The cortex is the outer region of a lymph node directly beneath the capsule.

Sinuses   Sinuses are irregular spaces through which the lymph percolates. The subcapsular sinus is the space between the capsule and the cortex; the peritrabecular sinuses surround the trabeculae. Macrophages span the sinuses; they phagocytize and destroy foreign materials (antigens) suspended in the lymph. Over 99% of the antigens entering a lymph node are destroyed by macrophages.

Primary Follicle   Aggregation of B cells and follicular dendritic cells.

Resting (inactive) B Cells   Most of the cells in primary follicles are resting (inactive) B cells. Follicular dendritic cells trap antigens encountered in the lymph and present them to B cells.

Secondary Follicle   (contains a germinal center) When activated by antigens, B cells migrate to the center of the follicle, forming a germinal center. Germinal centers are the central regions of secondary follicles where activated B cells are proliferating (dividing by mitosis) and differentiating into plasma cells and memory B cells. When stimulated by antigens, lymph nodes enlarge due to the formation of germinal centers and B cell proliferation.

Activated B Cells   Activated B cells enlarge, divide mitotically, and differentiate into plasma cells and memory B cells. Memory cells are found in the mantle zone (outer border of secondary follicle). Some B cells do not differentiate into plasma cells; they become memory B cells. Memory cells flow with the lymph and re-enter the blood circulatory system.

PARACORTICAL REGION

The paracortical region is between the cortex and the medulla.

Resting (inactive) T Cells   Resting T cells reside in the paracortical region. Interdigitating dendritic cells in the paracortical region trap antigens and present them to T cells.

MEDULLA

The medulla is the innermost portion of a lymph node adjacent to the hilus.

Medullary Sinuses   The lymph from cortical sinuses passes through the medullary sinuses and then exits the lymph node via the efferent lymphatic vessels.

Activated T Cells and Plasma Cells   Medullary cords (regions of densely packed lymphocytes) are composed of activated T cells and plasma cells.

FUNCTION

Nodes filter the lymph, removing foreign material and microorganisms (bacteria). All lymph is filtered by at least one lymph node before it returns to the blood. Antibody-mediated and cell-mediated immune responses occur in the lymph nodes.

LYMPH NODE

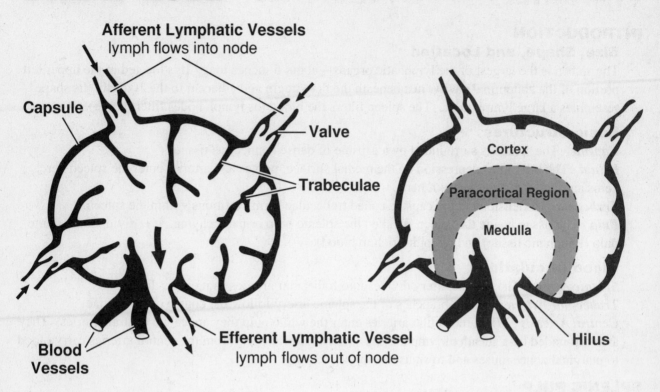

Afferent Lymphatic Vessels
lymph flows into node

Capsule

Valve

Trabeculae

Blood Vessels

Efferent Lymphatic Vessel
lymph flows out of node

Cortex

Paracortical Region

Medulla

Hilus

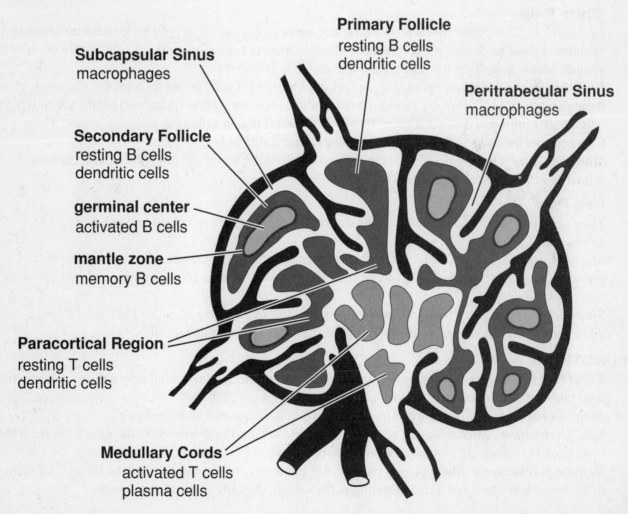

Primary Follicle
resting B cells
dendritic cells

Subcapsular Sinus
macrophages

Peritrabecular Sinus
macrophages

Secondary Follicle
resting B cells
dendritic cells

germinal center
activated B cells

mantle zone
memory B cells

Paracortical Region
resting T cells
dendritic cells

Medullary Cords
activated T cells
plasma cells

LYMPHATIC TISSUES / Spleen

INTRODUCTION
Size, Shape, and Location
The spleen is the largest of the lymphatic organs—about 5 inches long. It is located in the upper left portion of the abdominal cavity, just beneath the diaphragm and adjacent to the 10th rib. Its shape resembles a large lymph node. The spleen filters the blood (as lymph nodes filter lymph).

Basic Structures
Capsule   The spleen is surrounded by a capsule of dense connective tissue.
Hilum   The hilum is a depression on the medial surface; nerves and arteries enter the spleen here; veins and lymphatic vessels exit here.
Trabeculae   Extensions of the capsule called trabeculae form partitions within the spleen.
Pulp   The tissue inside the spleen is called the splenic pulp or parenchyma. It is divided into white pulp (lymphatic tissue) and red pulp (rich in blood).

Blood Circulation
Splenic Artery   The splenic artery divides into trabecular arteries as it enters the hilum.
Trabecular Arteries   These branches of the splenic artery follow the course of trabeculae.
Central Arteries   When trabecular arteries enter the white pulp they are called central arteries. They are surrounded by a sheath of lymphocytes. Arterioles branching from the central arteries carry blood to marginal zone sinuses and to sinusoids in the red pulp.

SPLENIC PULP
White Pulp
Periarteriolar Lymphatic Sheaths (PALS)   The white pulp consists of lymphatic tissue arranged in cylindrical sheaths (periarteriolar lymphatic sheaths) around central arteries.   T cells are found in greatest concentrations in the region closest to the central arteries.
Follicles (also called splenic nodules)   Spherical clusters of B cells called follicles are scattered throughout the PALS. Primary (unstimulated) follicles contain resting (inactive) B cells; secondary (stimulated) follicles contain activated B cells in a central region called the germinal center. These follicles have the same structural organization as those found in lymph nodes.
Marginal Zone   The marginal zone is the region between the white and red pulp. It is composed primarily of macrophages and dendritic cells.

Red Pulp
The red pulp is mainly concerned with the destruction of worn-out red blood cells. It consists of splenic cords and sinusoids.
Splenic Cords (Billroth's Cords)   Splenic cords consist of all cells between the sinusoids in the red pulp: reticular cells, macrophages, monocytes, lymphocytes, plasma cells, granulocytes, red blood cells, and platelets.
Sinusoids   Sinusoids are blood-filled spaces located throughout the red pulp. They have large, dilated, irregular lumens and large pores (spaces between the endothelial cells).

FUNCTIONS
Blood Cell Production   Lymphocytes produced in white pulp migrate to red pulp sinuses. During the fetal phase of development, granulocytes and erythrocytes are produced.
Blood Storage   A small quantity of blood is stored in the sinusoids of the red pulp.
RBC Destruction   Most worn-out or damaged red blood cells are destroyed in the spleen (some in the bone marrow). They are phagocytized by macrophages.
Defense Mechanisms   Macrophages phagocytize microbes that have penetrated the blood. Antigens in the blood activate B and T cells residing in the spleen, triggering immune responses.

SPLEEN (schematic)

The spleen filters the blood. The main function of the spleen is the phagocytosis of bacteria and worn-out or damaged red blood cells.

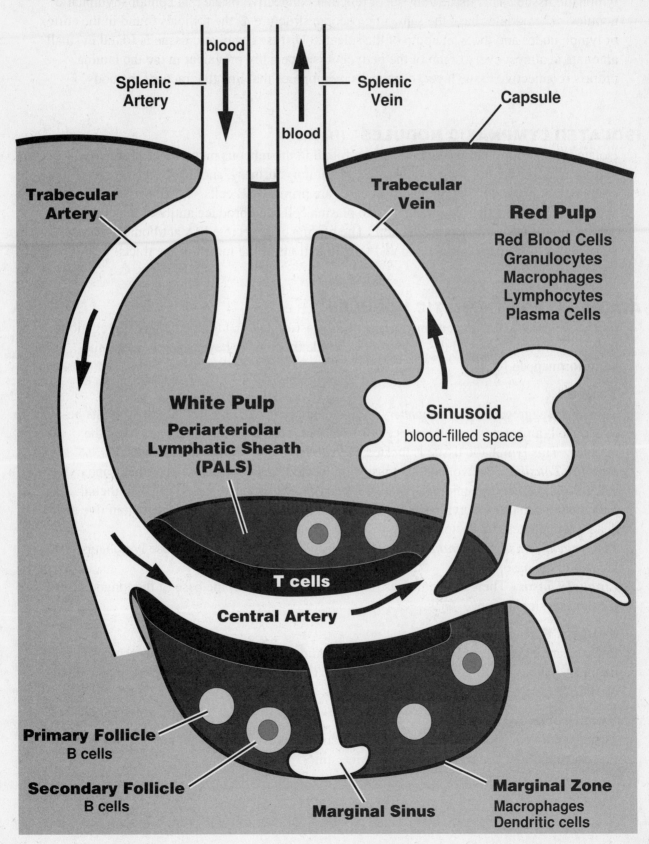

Splenic Artery

blood

blood

Splenic Vein

Capsule

Trabecular Artery

Trabecular Vein

Red Pulp

Red Blood Cells
Granulocytes
Macrophages
Lymphocytes
Plasma Cells

White Pulp

Periarteriolar Lymphatic Sheath (PALS)

Sinusoid
blood-filled space

T cells

Central Artery

Primary Follicle
B cells

Secondary Follicle
B cells

Marginal Sinus

Marginal Zone
Macrophages
Dendritic cells

LYMPHATIC TISSUES / Diffuse Lymphatic Tissue

When lymphatic tissue is not enclosed by a capsule, it is called diffuse or unencapsulated lymphatic tissue. This tissue consists of reticular connective tissue that contains lymphatic nodules. The nodules have the same microscopic structure as the follicles found in the cortex of lymph nodes and the white pulp of the spleen. Diffuse lymphatic tissue is found in small amounts in almost every organ of the body, but is especially prevalent in the the lamina propria (connective tissue layer) of mucous membranes that line the tracts of the body.

ISOLATED LYMPHATIC NODULES (B cells)

Isolated (individual) lymphatic nodules are found in the mucous membranes lining the various tracts of the body (gastrointestinal, respiratory, urinary, and reproductive tracts). The lymphocytes present in the lymphatic nodules are primarily B cells. When activated by the appropriate antigen, they differentiate into plasma cells and produce antibodies against the antigen that stimulated their production. The plasma cells secrete IgA antibodies, which provide protection against bacterial and viral infections in the lumen of the tracts.

AGGREGATED LYMPHATIC NODULES (B cells)

In certain regions, the mucous membrane of the gastrointestinal tract contains aggregations (clusters) of lymphatic nodules. Examples include the tonsils, Peyer's patches, and the vermiform appendix.

Tonsils

Tonsils are aggregates of *incompletely* encapsulated lymphatic tissue. A barrier exists between the lymphatic tissue and adjacent tissues, but it does not completely envelop the nodules. This lymphatic tissue is located beneath the epithelium of the pharynx.
Palatine Tonsils The two palatine tonsils are located in the lateral walls of the oropharynx. The tonsils consist of numerous lymphatic nodules. Each tonsil has 10 to 20 epithelial invaginations that form crypts (spaces) in the lymphatic tissue. The crypts contain live and dead lymphocytes and bacteria.
Pharyngeal Tonsil or *Adenoids* The pharyngeal tonsil is an area of diffuse lymphatic tissue located in the nasopharynx.
Lingual Tonsils There are numerous lingual tonsils located at the base of the tongue. Each tonsil has a single crypt.

Peyer's Patches

Peyer's patches are unencapsulated lymphatic nodules found in the lamina propria of the ileum (the lower portion of the small intestine). There are about 30 patches, each consisting of 10 to 200 nodules.

Vermiform Appendix

The appendix contains aggregations of lymphatic nodules. It is located on the cecum, the first portion of the ascending colon (large intestine).

DIFFUSE LYMPHATIC TISSUE

When lymphatic tissue is not enclosed by a capsule, it is called diffuse or unencapsulated lymphatic tissue.
Unencapsulated lymphatic nodules are found isolated or aggregated in the lining of the digestive, respiratory, urinary, and reproductive tracts.

Tonsils

Tonsils are aggregations of large lymphatic nodules embedded in the mucous membranes of the throat.

They form a ring of lymphatic tissue at the junction of the mouth cavity and pharynx (throat).

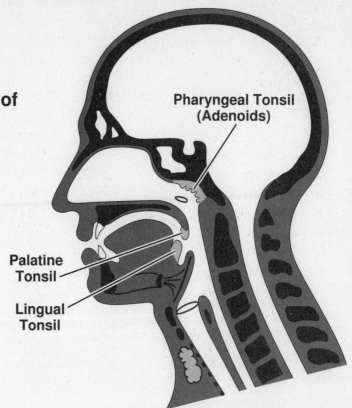

Pharyngeal Tonsil (Adenoids)

Palatine Tonsil

Lingual Tonsil

Tonsil (detail)

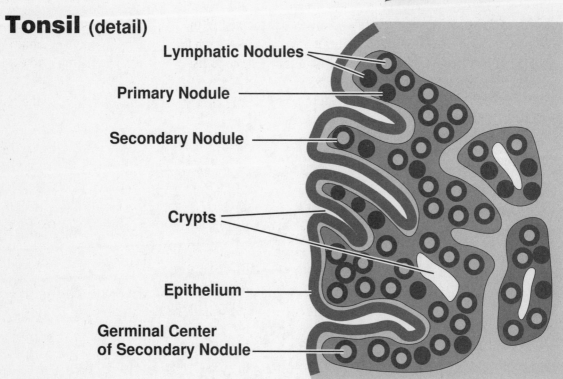

Lymphatic Nodules

Primary Nodule

Secondary Nodule

Crypts

Epithelium

Germinal Center of Secondary Nodule

41

4 Immune (Specific) Responses

IMMUNE RESPONSES / Overview

The sick were tended by the pitying care of those who had recovered, because they were themselves free of apprehension. For no one was ever attacked a second time.
— Thucydides (writing of the plague that swept Athens during the Peloponnesian War)

The words of Thucydides, written about 2500 years ago, show an understanding of the central concept of immunity: once exposed to a disease, the body adapts and becomes more resistant to that specific disease.

THE GERM THEORY

At the time of the Peloponnesian War it was not known that diseases were caused by microorganisms. In fact, microorganisms were not discovered until late in the 17th century by Anton van Leeuwenhoek; and they were not recognized as the cause of disease for another 200 years. The relationship between micro-organisms and disease became clear in the late 19th century largely through the work of the French chemist Louis Pasteur and the German bacteriologist Robert Koch: Pasteur studied disease in silkworms; Koch studied anthrax in sheep and tuberculosis in humans.

MEDICAL PROTECTION   (against specific infectious diseases)
Vaccination

In 1796 the British physician Edward Jenner discovered vaccination. He observed that milkmaids who had been infected with cowpox were protected from the more serious disease called smallpox. Edward Jenner inoculated healthy people with cowpox and found that they were protected from smallpox. This form of immunization was called vaccination because the Latin word for cowpox is *vaccinia* (*vacca* = cow). Now it is known that the protein coat of the cowpox virus is similar to that of the smallpox virus. The presence in the body of the cowpox protein stimulates the production of antibodies that are effective against both viruses.

Antibiotics

In 1929 the British bacteriologist Alexander Fleming discovered the first antibiotic, penicillin, although its effects were not reported until 1940. Penicillin is produced by the mold Penicillium, which grows on decaying fruits and ripening cheese; it inhibits the growth of various types of bacteria. Originally it was believed that antiboiotics could be produced only by living organisms; today many antibiotics, including penicillin, are synthesized in the laboratory.   Another example of an antibiotic is streptomycin.

Sulfa Drugs

In 1935 another "wonder drug" was discovered in Germany; it was sulfanilamide, a sulfur-containing organic compound that was capable of inhibiting the growth and activity of various kinds of bacteria. Other examples of sulfa drugs are sulfathiazole and sulfadiazine. Both sulfa drugs and penicillin were put into widespread use during World War II.

IMMUNE RESPONSES   (the body's methods of fighting specific infectious diseases)

An immune response is an altered reactivity to a specific antigen following contact with it.

Criteria   There are two main criteria for immune responses:

(1) Specificity : The altered response must be selective; only one type of bacterium, virus, or pollen grain is able to trigger the response.

(2) Memory : When a second infection occurs by the same type of virus or bacterium, the defense responses will be faster, so tissue damage will be minor.

Self vs. Nonself   Usually immunity to a specific substance will occur only if that substance is not found in the body; the immune system discriminates between "self" and "nonself." The exception is autoimmune diseases; the immune system attacks specific tissues of the body.

Mechanisms

(1) Antibody-Mediated Immunity (Humoral Immunity)   Specificity depends on antibodies.

(2) Cell-Mediated Immunity (Cellular Immunity)   Specificity depends on T cells.

IMMUNIZATIONS
(Vaccinations against infectious diseases)

Disease	Comments
Cholera	Present in the Middle East and Asia; 2 injections (2 to 6 weeks apart); booster shots every 6 months
Diptheria	Given in a series of 4 shots; booster shot every 7–10 years
Haemophilus Type B	Recommended for all children 2 years old
Hepatitis B	For people who do not test positive for antibodies to the hepatitis B virus and are at risk of acquiring the disease
Influenza	For the elderly and others at high risk of serious illness
Measles	Should be given to children at age 15 months; inoculation is usually combined: measles-mumps-rubella
Meningococcal Meningitis	Prevalent in regions of Africa and South America; types of vaccine : A, C, W-135, and Y
Mumps	Should be given to children at age 15 months; inoculation is usually combined: measles-mumps-rubella
Pertussis (Whooping Cough)	Begun between 1 and 3 months of age; usually combined with tetanus and diptheria; should not be given to children over 6 years of age
Plague	3 injections (one month or more apart)
Pneumococcal Pneumonia	For elderly people before traveling; one dose only (3 weeks before departure); no further doses should be given
Polio	Vaccine given orally at 2, 4, and 18 months of age; adults should also be immunized
Rabies	Common in domestic animals in India & South America; 3 injections at intervals of one week; booster injection 3 weeks later
Rubella	Should be given to children at age 15 months; inoculation is usually combined: measles-mumps-rubella
Smallpox	Smallpox has been eradicated as of 1980; no vaccination is now needed.
Tetanus	A series of shots completed by school age; a booster shot every 7 to 10 years for children over 12 and adults
Typhoid	2 doses (at least one month apart); booster shot every 3 years

IMMUNE RESPONSES / Antigens

DEFINITIONS

Antigen : any substance that, when introduced into the body, is recognized as foreign.

Endogenous Antigen : an antigen that originates inside the body. Examples of endogenous antigens are the proteins that are expressed on the outer surfaces of cancer cells and virus-infected cells; they are recognized as foreign by cytotoxic T cells.

Exogenous Antigens : an antigen that originates outside the body; recognized by helper T cells.

Antigen Receptor : a protein molecule located on the surface of a lymphocyte (B cell or T cells) that binds to a specific antigen.

Immunogenicity : the ability of an antigen to provoke an immune response.

Reactivity : the ability of an antigen to bind (react with) specific antibodies.

ANTIGEN STRUCTURE AND FUNCTION

Size and Composition Antigens are large, complex molecules. Molecular weight: 10,000 daltons or more. Antigens are usually protein (nucleo-, lipo-, or glycoprotein). Some large polysaccharides can be antigens. Entire microbes (bacteria or viruses) or parts of microbes can be antigens. Examples of nonmicrobial antigens include pollen, egg white, tissue transplants, or incompatible blood.

Antigenic Determinant (Epitope) An antigenic determinant is the site on an antigen molecule to which an antibody or T cell antigen receptor (TCR) binds by noncovalent interactions. The number of different antigenic determinants in the external environment is enormous (at least 1 billion). Each type of antigenic determinant has a different shape; and for each type of antigenic determinant there are a small number of lymphocytes ready and waiting that can recognize and respond to it. Each type of antigenic determinant induces the production of a different type of antibody or T cell, which mediates the elimination of the antigen.

Hapten (Partial Antigen) A hapten is a substance that is too small to function as an antigen, but when attached to a carrier molecule, it triggers an immune response. An example is the lipid toxin in poison ivy, which triggers an immune response after combining with a body protein. Hapten-stimulated immune responses are responsible for allergic reactions to drugs (such as penicillin) and other chemicals in the environment.

MAJOR HISTOCOMPATIBILITY COMPLEX PROTEINS (MHC Proteins)

MHC proteins are also called *MHC antigens* or *MHC molecules*. MHC proteins are a group of proteins found on the plasma membranes of all cells with a nucleus (red blood cells have no nuclei and no MHC proteins). They play an important role in cell-mediated immune responses : in order for a T cell to recognize an antigen, the antigen must be associated with an MHC protein.

They were named MHC proteins because the group of genes that codes for them is known as the major histocompatibility complex (MHC). No two individulals (except identical twins) have the same MHC genes, so no two individuals have the same MHC proteins. They are also called *human leukocyte-associated antigens (HLAs)*, because they were first identified on leukocytes. MHC proteins are the reason that transplanted tissues are rejected : the body recognizes the MHC antigens on the transplanted cells as foreign; T cells attack and kill the transplanted graft cells.

There are two categories of MHC proteins: class I and class II.

Class I MHC Proteins (MHC-I) MHC-I proteins are located on the surfaces of most body cells; endogenous antigens usually associate with MHC-I proteins. Cytotoxic T cells require antigen to be associated with MHC-I.

Class II MHC Proteins (MHC-II) MHC-II proteins are located on the surfaces of antigen presenting cells (macrophages, dendritic cells, and some B cells); exogenous antigens associate with MHC-II proteins. Helper T cells require antigen to be associated with MHC-II.

ANTIGENS

Antigens are molecules that are recognized as foreign .
Bacterial cells, virus-infected cells, cancer cells,
and the cells of disease-causing organisms
all have antigens that allow the body to recognize them as foreign.

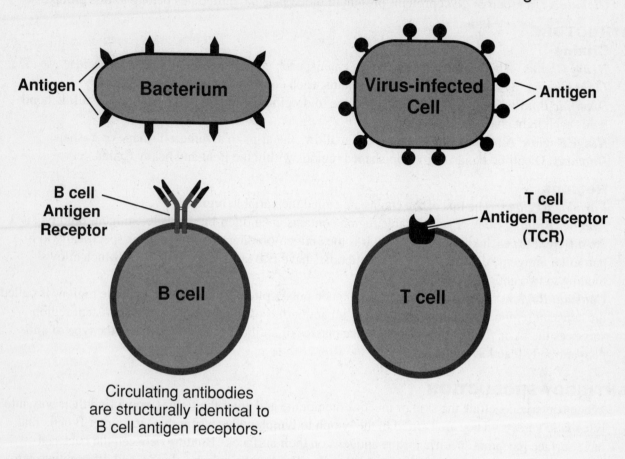

Circulating antibodies
are structurally identical to
B cell antigen receptors.

Antigenic Determinants (Epitopes)

A given antibody binds to a particular part of its antigen
called the antigenic determinant (or epitope).

Most antigen molecules have several different antigenic determinants.

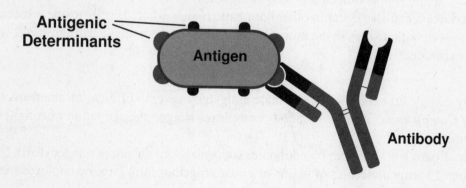

IMMUNE RESPONSES / Antibodies

DEFINITIONS

Antibody (Ab) : a protein that combines with the antigenic determinant that triggered its production.
Immunoglobulin (Ig) : another term for antibody.
Globulins : a group of glycoproteins present in blood plasma; antibodies belong to this group.

STRUCTURE
Chains

Heavy Chains There are 2 identical heavy chains; each consists of about 450 amino acids.
Light Chains There are 2 identical light chains; each consists of about 200 amino acids.
Disulfide Bonds Two disulfide bonds link the midregions of the heavy chains; one disulfide bond holds each light chain to a heavy chain.
Hinge Region A region on each heavy chain allows the arms to assume a T-shape or Y-shape.
Domains Disulfide bonds form loop-shaped regions within the light and heavy chains.

Regions

Variable Regions The tips of the chains are called the variable regions.
Antigen-Binding Sites Each variable region contains an antigen-binding site; antigen- binding sites are different for each kind of antibody. It is the antigen-binding site that attaches specifically to a particular antigenic determinant. Most antibodies have two antigen-binding sites, which allows binding to two antigenic determinants.
Constant Region The remaining portion of each polypeptide chain (less the variable region) is called the constant region. It is nearly the same in all antibodies of the same class. The constant region serves as the basis for distinguishing the five classes of antibodies, and determines the type of antigen–antibody reaction that occurs.

ANTIBODY PRODUCTION

When bacteria penetrate the skin or mucous membrane and enter the tissues, some find their way into lymphatic vessels. They are carried in the lymph to lymph nodes where they encounter B cells that have surface receptors specific for the antigens on their surfaces. Binding between the bacterial antigens and B cell receptors activates the B cells. The B cells enlarge, divide, and differentiate into plasma cells. Plasma cells are specialized to synthesize protein, so their cytoplasm is filled with an unusually large amount of rough endoplasmaic reticulum (the site of protein synthesis). Antibodies (proteins) that are capable of binding to the type of antigen that stimulated their production are synthesized and released from the plasma cells. They are carried out of the lymph node in the lymph and blood, and circulated to all parts of the body. When they encounter an antigen that matches their binding sites, they bind, forming antigen-antibody complexes.

Antibody production can also occur in other lymphatic tissues where B cells reside, especially the spleen and diffuse lymphatic tissues in the mucous membranes of the tracts (gastrointestinal, respiratory, urinary, and reproductive).

FUNCTIONS

Antigen-antibody complexes neutralize or eliminate antigen by several different mechanisms :
(1) Activation of Complement Antigen-antibody complexes trigger the activation of complement by the classical complement pathway .
(2) Phagocytosis Coating of microbes by antibodies (opsonization) enhances phagocytosis.
(3) Neutralization Linking molecules of toxins or viruses together form larger complexes that are no longer harmful to the body.

ANTIBODY STRUCTURE
The Basic Antibody (Immunoglobulin) Structure

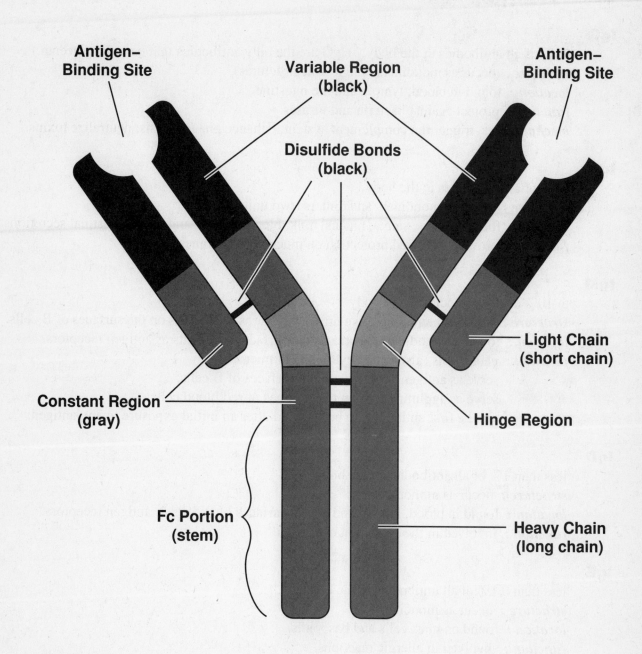

Antigen–
Binding Site

Variable Region
(black)

Antigen–
Binding Site

Disulfide Bonds
(black)

Light Chain
(short chain)

Constant Region
(gray)

Hinge Region

Fc Portion
(stem)

Heavy Chain
(long chain)

CLASSES OF ANTIBODIES

There are five different classes of antibodies (immunoglobulins). Each has a distinct chemical structure and a specific biological role.

IgG

75% of all antibodies in the body. (IgG are the only antibodies that pass the placenta.)

structure : occur as monomers (single unit structures).

location : found in blood, lymph, and the intestine.

function : protect against bacteria and viruses.

mechanisms : trigger the complement system; enhance phagocytosis; neutralize toxins.

IgA

15% of all antibodies in the body.

structure : occur as monomers and dimers (two units).

location : found in tears, saliva, mucus, milk, blood, lymph, and gastrointestinal secretions.

function : provide localized protection on mucous membranes.

IgM

5–10% of all antibodies in the body.

structure : occur as pentamers (five units). Occur as monomers on the surfaces of B cells.

location : found in blood, lymph, and on the surfaces of B cells as antigen receptors.

function : cause lysis (also called cytolysis) of microbes;
        serve as antigen receptors on the surfaces of B cells;
        serve as agglutinogens on the surfaces of red blood cells;
        are the first antibodies to be secreted after an initial exposure to any antigen.

IgD

less than 1% of all antibodies in the body.

structure : occur as monomers.

location : found in blood, lymph, and on the surfaces of B cells as antigen receptors.

function : involved in the activation of B cells.

IgE

less than 0.1% of all antibodies in the body.

structure : occur as monomers.

location : found on mast cells and basophils.

function : involved in allergic reactions.

ANTIBODY CLASSIFICATION

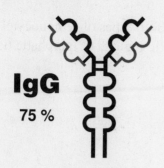

IgG
75 %

FUNCTIONS :

protects against bacteria and viruses
by
enhancing phagocytosis
neutralizing toxins
triggering the complement system

IgA
15 %

FUNCTIONS :

provide localized protection
on mucous membranes

IgM
5 - 10 %

FUNCTIONS :

cause agglutination and lysis of microbes

serve as antigen receptors for B cells
(present as monomers on surfaces of B cells)

involved in the agglutination of blood
during transfusions

IgD
1 %

FUNCTION :

involved in the
activation of B cells

IgE
0.1 %

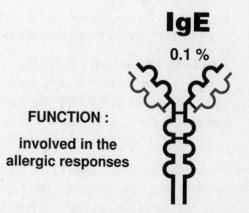

FUNCTION :

involved in the
allergic responses

51

IMMUNE RESPONSES / Lymphocytes

There are two basic types of lymphocytes: B cells and T cells. Both types of lymphocytes differentiate from stem cells in the bone marrow and migrate to specific regions of lymphatic tissues, where they wait to be activated by their antigens.

B CELLS : ORIGIN AND MATURATION
Stem Cells
Stem cells in the bone marrow differentiate into mature B cells.

Mature B Cells
Mature B cells migrate via the blood to lymphatic tissues: diffuse lymphatic tissue in the mucous membranes of tracts (including the tonsils), lymph nodes, and spleen.

Resting (inactive) B Cells
Diffuse Lymphatic Tissue (Tonsils) In diffuse lymphatic tissues *lymphatic nodules* (structurally the same as primary follicles found in lymph nodes and spleen) contain resting B cells.
Lymph Nodes Resting B cells form *primary follicles (lymphatic nodules)* in the cortex of lymph nodes.
Spleen In the spleen, resting B cells form *primary follicles (splenic nodules)* in the white pulp.

The mature resting B cells in the diffuse lymphatic tissues, lymph nodes, and spleen remain inactive until they are stimulated by the appropriate antigens. For every type of antigen there are a small number of B cells that have surface receptors that can bind to them ("recognize" them).

T CELLS : ORIGIN AND MATURATION
Stem Cells
Stem cells in the bone marrow differentiate into immature T cells.

Immature T Cells
Immature T cells migrate from the bone marrow to the thymus gland via the blood.
In the thymus, immature T cells divide and differentiate into 3 subsets of mature T cells: helper T cells, cytotoxic T cells, and suppressor T cells. Helper T cells and suppressor T cells acquire a surface protein called CD4; cytotoxic T cells acquire a surface protein called CD8. The T cells also acquire surface proteins that function as T cell antigen receptors (TCRs). There are millions of different T cells, each with unique TCRs.

Mature T Cells
The mature T cells (CD4+ T cells and CD8+ T cells) migrate from the thymus gland and travel via the blood to thymus-dependent areas of the lymph nodes and spleen.

Resting (inactive) T Cells
Lymph Nodes Mature T cells aggregate in the paracortical region (middle region) of lymph nodes. These mature T cells are called resting or inactive T cells.
Spleen In the spleen, mature T cells form a sheath around the central arteries. This region is called the periarteriolar lymphatic sheath (PALS).

The mature resting T cells in the lymph nodes and spleen remain inactive until they are stimulated by the appropriate antigens. For every type of antigen there are a small number of T cells that have surface receptors that can bind to them ("recognize" them).

LYMPHOCYTES
Origin, Maturation, and Locations in Lymphatic Tissues

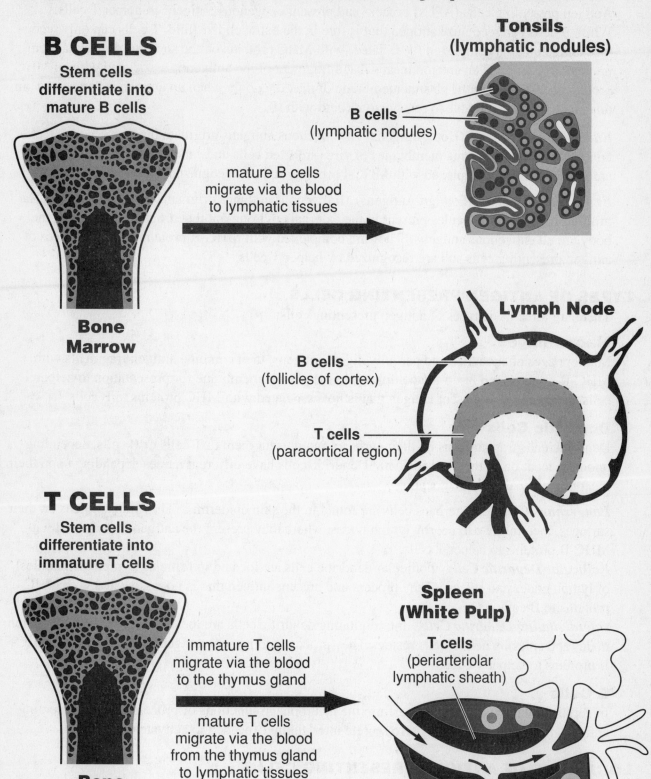

B CELLS

Stem cells differentiate into mature B cells

mature B cells migrate via the blood to lymphatic tissues

Bone Marrow

Tonsils (lymphatic nodules)

B cells (lymphatic nodules)

Lymph Node

B cells (follicles of cortex)

T cells (paracortical region)

T CELLS

Stem cells differentiate into immature T cells

immature T cells migrate via the blood to the thymus gland

mature T cells migrate via the blood from the thymus gland to lymphatic tissues

Bone Marrow

Spleen (White Pulp)

T cells (periarteriolar lymphatic sheath)

B cells (follicles)

IMMUNE RESPONSES / Antigen Presenting Cells (APCs)

Antigen presenting cells (APCs) process and present exogenous antigens to helper T cells. While B cells can recognize antigen that is free in the extracellular fluid, T cells can only recognize antigen that is complexed (associated) with MHC proteins on the surfaces of plasma membranes. "Presenting" an antigen means that a fragment of the antigen is associated with an MHC protein and inserted in the plasma membrane of the APC; only when an antigen is "presented" in this manner is a T cell able to recognize it (bind with it).

Endogenous Antigens (Host Antigens) Endogenous antigens originate inside the body. Certain proteins on the plasma membranes of virus-infected cells and cancer cells are endogenous antigens. They are complexed with MHC-I proteins and are recognized by cytotoxic T cells.

Exogenous Antigens (Foreign Antigens) Exogenous antigens originate outside the body. The millions of protein molecules present in the external environment that are not produced by the body are all exogenous antigens. They are complexed with MHC-II proteins on the surfaces of antigen presenting cells and are recognized by helper T cells.

TYPES OF ANTIGEN PRESENTING CELLS

There are three basic types of antigen presenting cells:

Macrophages

Macrophages phagocytize and partially digest antigens; then combine antigen fragments with MHC-II proteins and insert the complex into the plasma membrane for presentation to helper T cells. They can also present antigen that is not associated with MHC proteins to B cells.

Dendritic Cells

Dendritic cells trap antigens on their surfaces and present them to T cells or B cells, depending upon the location of the dendritic cell. Dendritic cells have different names depending upon their locations; they are not phagocytic.

Langerhans Cells Langerhans cells are found in the skin epidermis. They trap antigens on their surfaces, then migrate to nearby lymph nodes, where they present the antigens complexed with MHC-II proteins to helper T cells.

Follicular Dendritic Cells Follicular dendritic cells are located in follicles (lymphatic nodules) of lymph nodes and spleen. They process and present antigen that is not associated with MHC proteins to B cells.

Interdigitating Dendritic Cells Interdigitating dendritic cells are located in the regions of lymph nodes and spleen where T cells reside. They process and present antigen complexed with MHC-II proteins to helper T cells.

B Cells

In certain situations B cells can perform the macrophage functions of processing and presenting antigens to helper T cells; they also secrete interleukin-1 (needed to activate the T cells).

LOCATIONS OF ANTIGEN PRESENTING CELLS

Antigen presenting cells are found in four basic locations: skin epidermis, diffuse lymphatic tissue (mucous membranes of tracts), lymph nodes, and spleen.

ANTIGEN PRESENTING CELLS

Antigen Presenting Cells Process and Present Antigens to
Helper T Cells and B Cells.

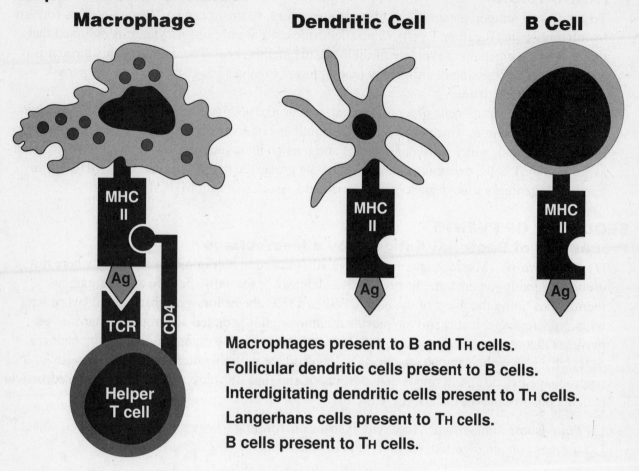

Macrophage   **Dendritic Cell**   **B Cell**

Macrophages present to B and T$_H$ cells.

Follicular dendritic cells present to B cells.

Interdigitating dendritic cells present to T$_H$ cells.

Langerhans cells present to T$_H$ cells.

B cells present to T$_H$ cells.

Locations of Antigen Presenting Cells

Macrophages are found in many tissues of the body.
Dendritic cells are found in the skin (Langerhans cells)
and in lymphatic tissues (follicular dendritic cells and
interdigitating dendritic cells). B cells are found in lymphatic tissues.

Lymph Node

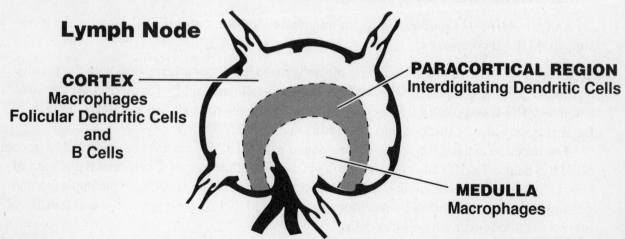

CORTEX
Macrophages
Folicular Dendritic Cells
and
B Cells

PARACORTICAL REGION
Interdigitating Dendritic Cells

MEDULLA
Macrophages

INTRODUCTION

To process an antigen means to modify it in some way, so that it can be "recognized" as foreign by a lymphocyte (B cell or T cell). Since dendritic cells are not phagocytic, it is assumed that they process antigen on the surface of their plasma membranes. The details of this mechanism are not clear. Processing of antigen by macrophages involves phagocytosis and the partial digestion of the antigens.

Antigen presenting cells process both exogenous and endogenous antigens. A macrophage phagocytizes bacteria, which have exogenous antigens on their surfaces, and virus-infected cells (and cancer cells), which have endogenous antigens on their surfaces. In order to be recognized as foreign by T cells, exogenous antigens must be processed and associated with MHC-II proteins; endogenous antigens must be processed and associated with MHC-I proteins.

SEQUENCE OF EVENTS
Processing of Bacterial Antigens by a Macrophage

(1) Phagocytosis Macrophages are strategically located in all regions of the body where microbes are likely to penetrate the nonspecific defenses (especially the skin and the mucous membranes lining the tracts of the body). When a microbe or foreign substance makes contact with a macrophage, it sticks to the plasma membrane; this is called adherence. Microbes or particles that are opsonized (coated with IgG antibodies or C3b complement proteins) adhere especially well, enhancing phagocytosis. Upon contact with the microbe or foreign particle, the macrophage extends pseudopods that surround it and fuse, forming a membrane-enclosed vesicle called a phagosome (or phagocytic vesicle).

(2) Phagosome Phagosomes fuse with lysosomes, forming a vesicle called a phagolysosome. Lysosomes contain digestive (hydrolytic) enzymes.

(3) Phagolysosome Within the phagolysosome digestive enzymes split large protein molecules (antigens) into short peptides (antigen fragments).

MHC proteins combine with some of the antigen fragments. There are different theories for explaining how the MHC proteins get into the phagolysosomes. One theory suggests that some of the MHC proteins already present on the surface of the macrophage at the time of endocytosis are included in the phagosome when it pinches off. (This is the mechanism illustrated on the facing page.) Another theory suggests that MHC proteins synthesized by smooth endoplasmic reticulum are packaged in Golgi vesicles, which fuse with the phagolysosome.

(4) Antigen–MHC-II Complex Antigen fragments combine with MHC-II proteins, forming antigen–MHC-II complexes.

(5) Exocytosis. The vesicles containing the antigen–MHC-II complexes fuse with the plasma membrane and the contents are released into the extracellular fluid by exocytosis. At this time antigen–MHC-II complexes are inserted into the plasma membrane. Uncomplexed antigen fragments may also be inserted into the plasma membrane.

The bacterial antigen fragments that associate with MHC-II proteins are presented to (recognized by) helper T cells (T4 cells), triggering activation of the helper T cells and the release of lymphokines such as interleukin-2 (IL-2), which helps to activate B cells. Uncomplexed antigen fragments are recognized by receptors on B cells, triggering their activation and transformation into antibody-secreting plasma cells.

ANTIGEN PROCESSING
Example: A Macrophage Processing Bacterial Antigens

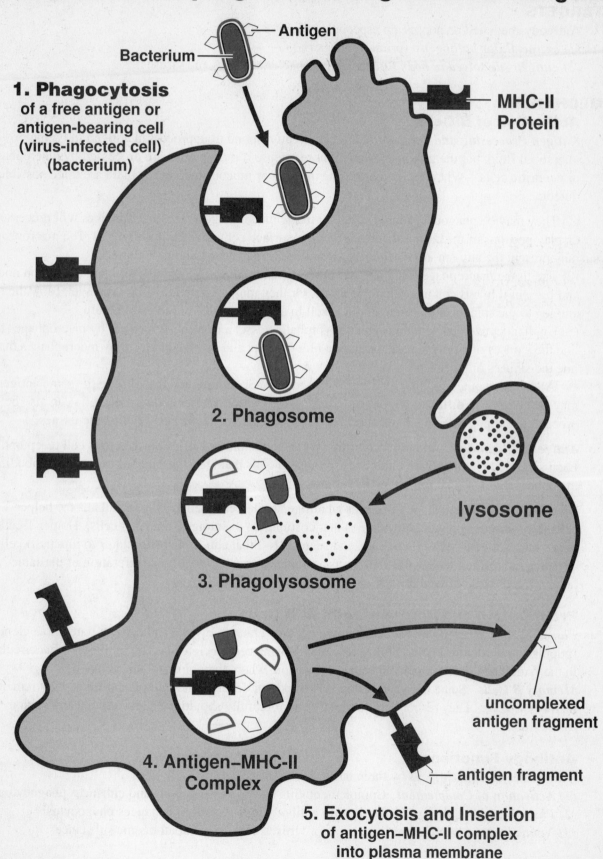

Antigen

Bacterium

1. Phagocytosis
of a free antigen or
antigen-bearing cell
(virus-infected cell)
(bacterium)

MHC-II
Protein

2. Phagosome

3. Phagolysosome

lysosome

**4. Antigen–MHC-II
Complex**

uncomplexed
antigen fragment

antigen fragment

5. Exocytosis and Insertion
of antigen–MHC-II complex
into plasma membrane

IMMUNE RESPONSES / Antibody–Mediated Immunity

TARGETS
Antibody-mediated responses are especially effective against:
(1) extracellular pathogens (primarily bacteria).
(2) antigens dissolved in body fluids (such as bacterial toxins and viruses).

MECHANISM
Activation of B Cells

Antigen Processing and Presentation B cells can respond to unprocessed antigen in lymph or interstitial fluid, but the response is much more intense if the antigens are processed by macrophages or dendritic cells. When bacteria penetrate the skin or mucous membrane there are three possible outcomes:

(1) They may be phagocytized and killed by tissue macrophages. The macrophages will process and display portions of the bacterial antigen on their surface complexed with MHC-II. The macrophage may present the antigen–MHC-II complex to B cells in nearby lymphatic tissues.
(2) The tissue macrophages may migrate into a lymphatic vessel, carry the antigen to a lymph node, and present it to a B cell in a primary follicle. Or they may migrate into a blood vessel, carry the antigen to the spleen, and present it to a B cell in a follicle located in the white pulp.
(3) Unphagocytized bacteria may enter a lymphatic vessel and be phagocytized by macrophages that line the sinuses of a lymph node; or enter a blood vessel and be phagocytized by macrophages that line the sinuses of the spleen.

All of these outcomes may occur simultaneously. So an immune response to the same antigen may be initiated in different lymphatic tissues of the body at the same time. Bacteria can also be processed and presented by dendritic cells, which are located in the same lymphatic tissues.

Antigen Recognition Antigen recognition refers to the binding of an antigen to B cell receptors. Each specific type of antigen binds only to those B cells that are programmed to secrete antibodies that attack (bind to) that same type of antigen.

Costimulation Macrophages also present antigen to helper T cells. This stimulates the helper T cells to proiferate and secrete cytokines that costimulate the antigen-bound B cells. Helper T cells bind to the antigen–MHC-II complex and secrete IL-2 that acts as a costimulator to initiate B cell division and differentiation; IL-2 also acts as an autocrine, stimulating proliferation of the same helper T cells that secreted it.

Proliferation and Differentiation of B Cells
Plasma Cells When B cells become activated, they enlarge, divide, and differentiate into a clone (population of identical cells) of plasma cells. Plasma cells secrete specific antibodies that circulate in the lymph and blood to reach the site of invasion, where they bind to their antigens.
Memory B Cells Some of the activated B cells do not differentiate into plasma cells; they remain as memory B cells. They respond more rapidly and forcefully should the same antigen appear at a future time.

Antibody Functions
Antibodies destroy antigens by three basic mechanisms:
(1) Activation of Complement Complement kills bacteria by cytolysis and enhances phagocytosis.
(2) Phagocytosis Coating of bacteria with antibody (opsonization) enhances phagocytosis.
(3) Neutralization Antibodies link toxins or viruses, forming nonpathogenic substances.

ANTIBODY–MEDIATED IMMUNITY

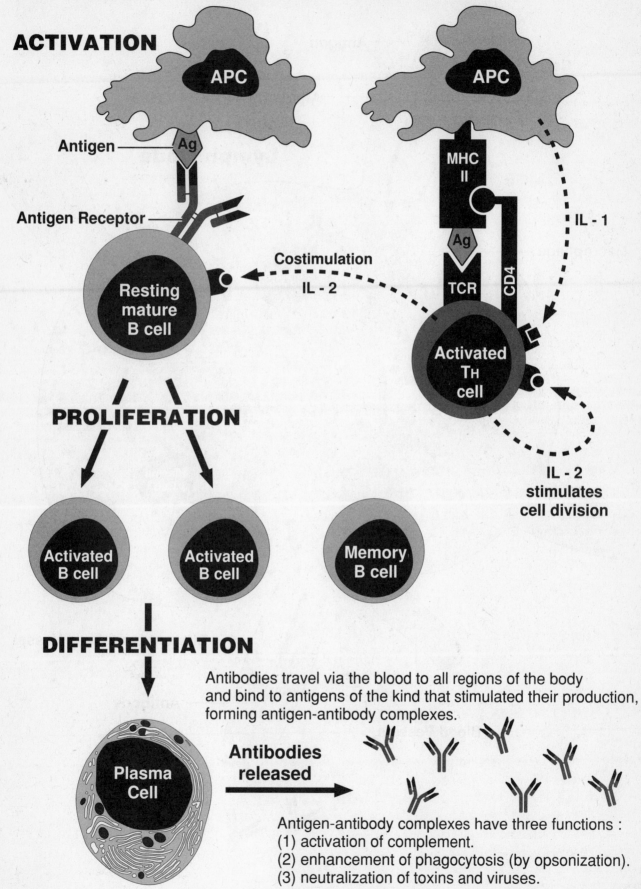

ACTIVATION

APC

Antigen — Ag

Antigen Receptor

Resting mature B cell

APC

MHC II

Ag

TCR   CD4

IL - 1

Costimulation
IL - 2

Activated TH cell

IL - 2 stimulates cell division

PROLIFERATION

Activated B cell

Activated B cell

Memory B cell

DIFFERENTIATION

Plasma Cell

Antibodies released

Antibodies travel via the blood to all regions of the body and bind to antigens of the kind that stimulated their production, forming antigen-antibody complexes.

Antigen-antibody complexes have three functions :
(1) activation of complement.
(2) enhancement of phagocytosis (by opsonization).
(3) neutralization of toxins and viruses.

ANTIBODY PRODUCTION IN LYMPH NODE

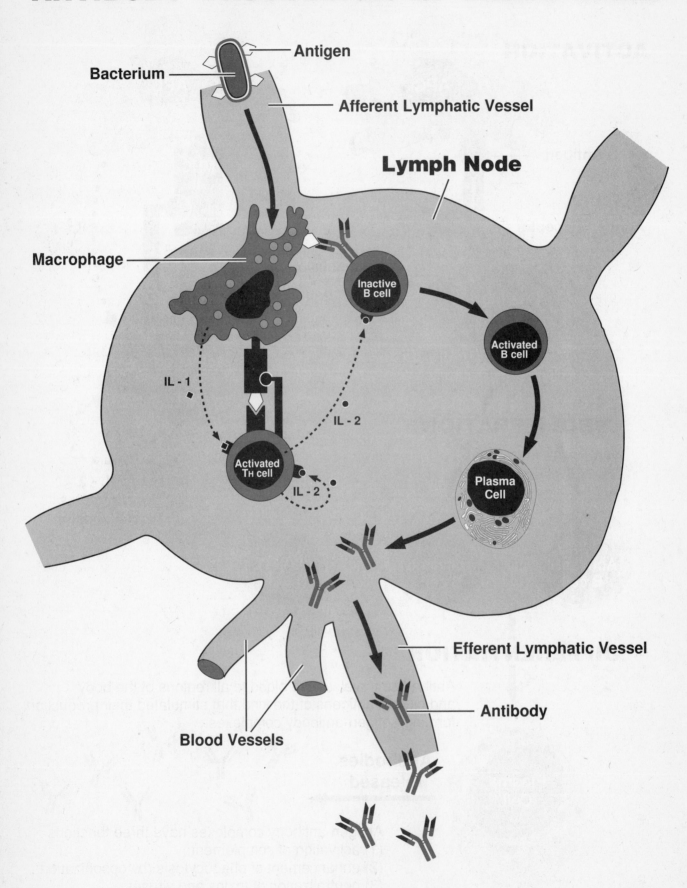

Bacterium

Antigen

Afferent Lymphatic Vessel

Lymph Node

Macrophage

IL - 1

Inactive B cell

Activated B cell

IL - 2

Activated TH cell

IL - 2

Plasma Cell

Efferent Lymphatic Vessel

Antibody

Blood Vessels

ANTIBODY FUNCTIONS

Activation of Complement

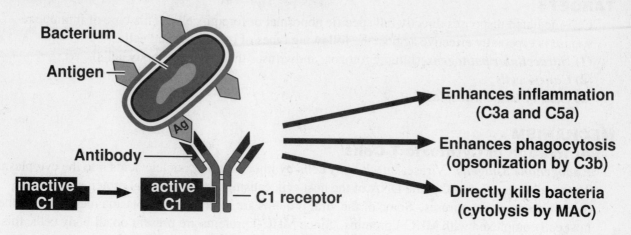

Bacterium

Antigen

Antibody

inactive C1 → active C1

C1 receptor

Enhances inflammation
(C3a and C5a)

Enhances phagocytosis
(opsonization by C3b)

Directly kills bacteria
(cytolysis by MAC)

Phagocytosis

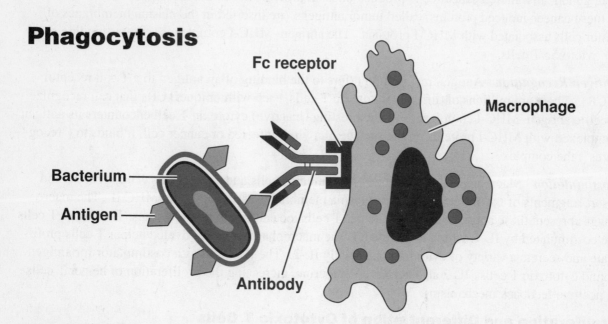

Fc receptor

Macrophage

Bacterium

Antigen

Antibody

Neutralization

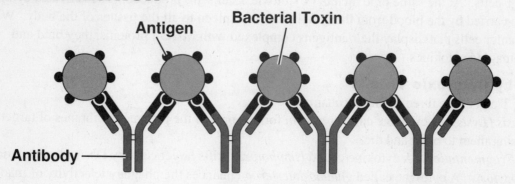

Antigen

Bacterial Toxin

Antibody

IMMUNE RESPONSES / Cell–Mediated Immunity

TARGETS

Cell-mediated responses directly kill specific abnormal or foreign cells. This type of immune response is especially effective against the following types of organisms and cells:

(1) Intracellular pathogens (fungi, protozoa, and viruses that are inside body cells).

(2) Cancer cells.

(3) Cells of tissue transplants.

MECHANISM

Activation of Cytotoxic T Cells

Endogenous Antigens Viruses attack body cells by injecting their nucleic acids into the cytoplasm. The viral nucleic acids alter the DNA of the host cell, causing it produce viral proteins, which are used to produce new viruses. Some of the viral proteins are inserted in the plasma membrane of the host cell complexed with MHC-I proteins. Since MHC-I proteins are present on all body cells, this type of antigen–MHC-I complex can be formed by any virus-infected cell.

Tumor Antigens Cancer cells result from genetic changes induced by viruses, chemicals, or radiation; genetically altered cancer cells produce unusual proteins not found in normal body cells. Some of these cancer-induced proteins, called tumor antigens, are inserted in the plasma membranes of tumor cells associated with MHC-I proteins. The antigen–MHC-I complexes serve as binding sites for cytotoxic T cells.

Antigen Recognition Antigen recognition refers to the binding of an antigen to a T cell receptor (TCR). There are millions of different cytotoxic T cells, each with unique TCRs that can recognize specific antigen–MHC-I complexes. When a resting (inactive) cytotoxic T cell encounters its antigen complexed with MHC-I proteins on the surface of a virus-infected or cancer cell, it binds to ("recognizes") the complex.

Costimulation Macrophages phagocytize virus-infected cells and cancer cells. They process and insert fragments of the antigens into their plasma membranes associated with MHC II. The macrophages present these antigens to resting helper T cells located in lymphatic tissues. The helper T cells are costimulated by IL-1, which is secreted by the macrophages. The activated helper T cells proliferate and secrete a variety of cytokines, especially IL-2. The IL-2 acts as a costimulator for antigen-bound cytotoxic T cells. IL-2 also acts as an autocrine, increasing the proliferation of helper T cells (a positive feedback mechanism).

Proliferation and Differentiation of Cytotoxic T Cells

Activated cytotoxic T cells enlarge and divide, forming a clone (population of identical cells) of cytotoxic T cells. At the same time memory cytotoxic T cells are produced. The activated cytotoxic T cells are carried by the blood from the lymph nodes or spleen to all the tissues of the body. When they encounter cells that display their antigens complexed with MHC-I proteins, they bind and release damaging cytokines.

Attack by Cytotoxic T Cells

Cytotoxic T cells have three killing mechanisms :

(1) Cytolysis (Lysis) A cytokine called *perforin* forms pores in the plasma membranes of target cells, causing them to burst and die.

(2) DNA Fragmentation A cytokine called *lymphotoxin* kills target cells by DNA fragmentation.

(3) Phagocytosis A cytokine called *gamma-interferon* enhances the phagocytic activity of macrophages, which ingest and kill the target cells.

CELL–MEDIATED IMMUNITY

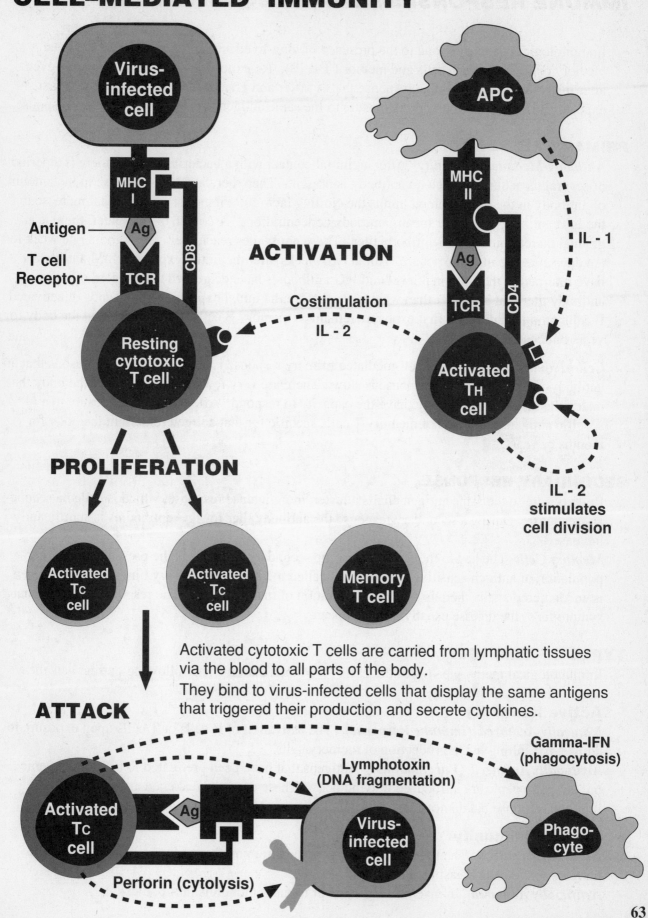

Virus-infected cell

APC

MHC I

MHC II

Antigen — Ag

ACTIVATION

T cell Receptor — TCR

CD8

Ag

TCR

CD4

IL - 1

Costimulation
IL - 2

Resting cytotoxic T cell

Activated T_H cell

IL - 2 stimulates cell division

PROLIFERATION

Activated T_C cell

Activated T_C cell

Memory T cell

Activated cytotoxic T cells are carried from lymphatic tissues via the blood to all parts of the body.

They bind to virus-infected cells that display the same antigens that triggered their production and secrete cytokines.

ATTACK

Gamma-IFN (phagocytosis)

Lymphotoxin (DNA fragmentation)

Activated T_C cell

Ag

Virus-infected cell

Phago-cyte

Perforin (cytolysis)

IMMUNE RESPONSES / Immunological Memory

Immunological memory is due to the presence of long-lived antibodies and very long-lived memory cells (memory B cells and memory T cells). Re-exposure to the same antigen—even after many years—calls forth a response that is faster and greater than the response to a first exposure. This response upon re-exposure to the same antigen is called the secondary response.

PRIMARY RESPONSE

Antibody-Mediated Immunity After an initial contact with a bacterial antigen, there is a period of several days during which no antibody is present. Then there is a slow increase in the amount of antibody in the serum (blood minus the clotting factors). First, there is a gradual increase in the IgM antibody titer (*titer* means antibody concentration). A couple of days later, there is a gradual increase in the IgG antibody titer. These antibodies reach their peaks about one week to ten days after the initial exposure. About two weeks after the initial exposure, IgM antibodies have returned to their original level and IgG antibodies have decreased and leveled off at an antibody titer that is greater than what it was before the initial exposure. Thousands of activated B cells produced during a first exposure remain as memory B cells, which remain in the body for years or decades.

Cell-Mediated Immunity A cell-mediated primary response is slow for the same reasons that an antibody-mediated primary response is slow. There are very few T cells present in the body that match the invading antigen and have the capacity to respond. After an initial exposure to a specific antigen, thousands of memory T cells specific for that antigen remain in the body for months or years.

SECONDARY RESPONSE

Re-exposure to the same antigen elicits a faster, more intense response, which is called a secondary response. During a secondary response the antibody titer for IgG antibodies is significantly increased.

Memory Cells The key to the quickness of the secondary response is the presence of a larger population of antigen-sensitive lymphocytes called memory cells. Every time the same antigen is encountered again, there is a rapid proliferation of memory cells. The response is so fast that symptoms of the disease usually do not appear.

TYPES OF IMMUNITY

Immunological memory provides the basis for immunization. The following outline lists the four basic types of immunity.

Active Immunity

Naturally Acquired (Immune Response) The activation of B cells or T cells upon exposure to antigens, resulting in the production of memory cells.

Artificially Acquired (Vaccinations) Antigens that have been pretreated to be immunogenic but not pathogenic are introduced into the body. These dead or weakened antigens cause an immune response but do not cause significant illness. Memory cells are produced.

Passive Immunity

Naturally Acquired The transfer of IgG antibodies from mother to fetus; or from mother to baby in milk during breast feeding.

Artificially Acquired Intravenous injection of immunoglobulins (antibodies).

PRIMARY AND SECONDARY RESPONSES

Primary Response (first exposure to a particular antigen)

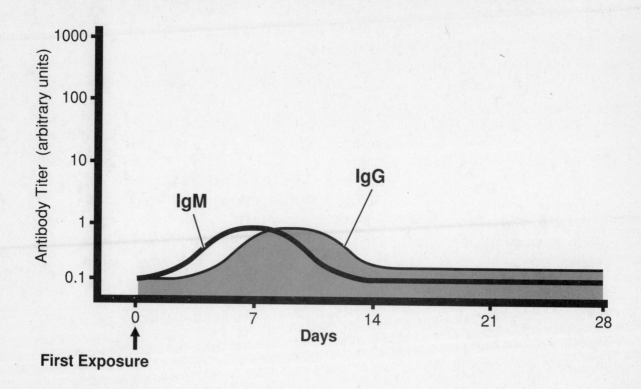

Secondary Response (second exposure to the same antigen)

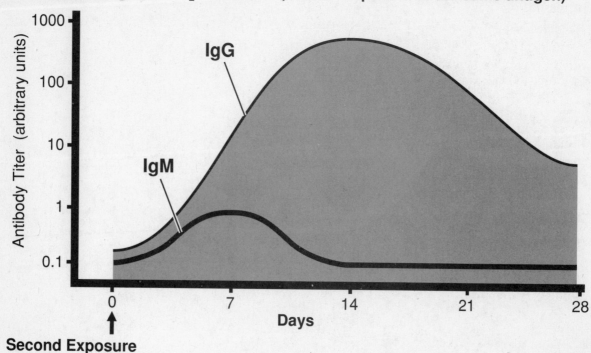

Part II : Self-Testing Exercises

Unlabeled illustrations from Part I

INFECTIONS
Infections arise when pathogens enter the body and multiply.

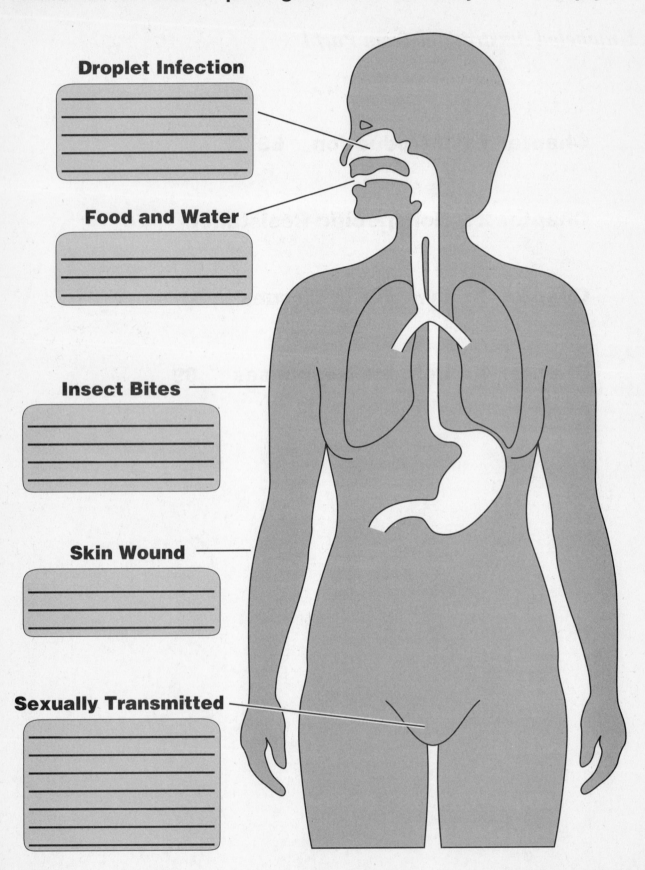

Droplet Infection

Food and Water

Insect Bites

Skin Wound

Sexually Transmitted

BACTERIA

The shapes of various bacteria as seen through a light microscope

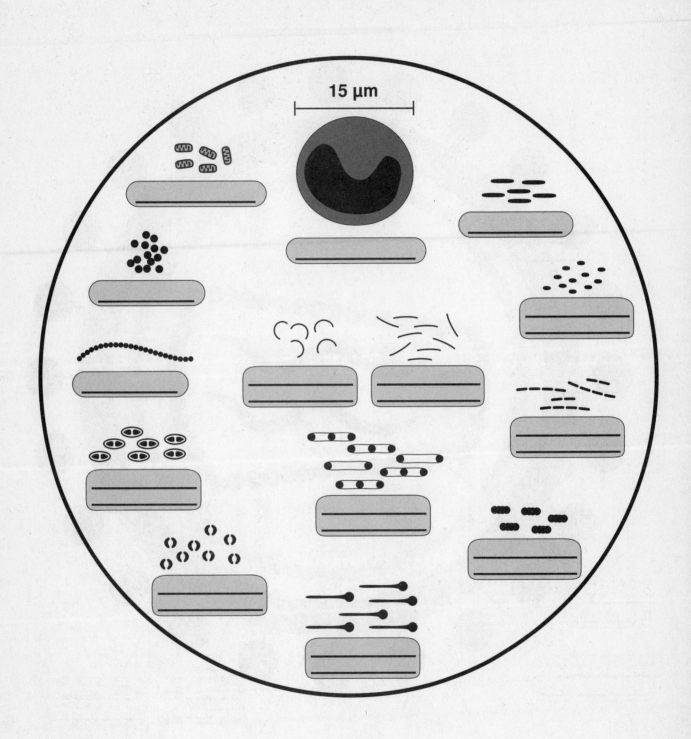

VIRUSES

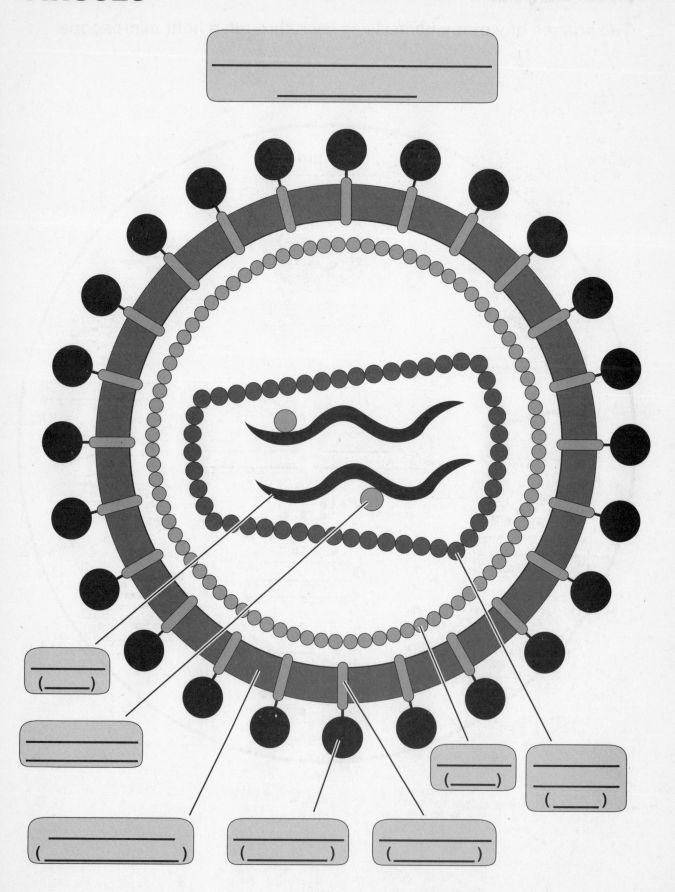

PARASITES
Tapeworm (Taenia saginata)

Head (_____)   Segment (_____)

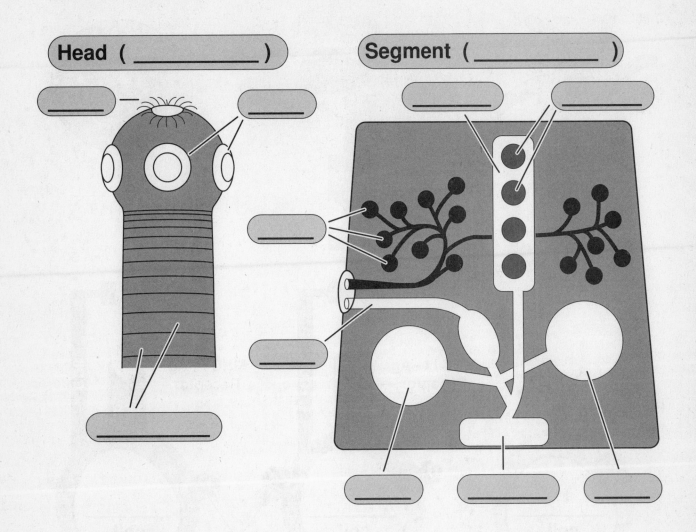

Human Intestine

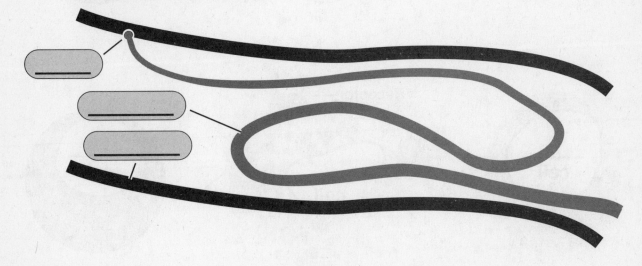

TYPES OF EFFECTOR CELLS

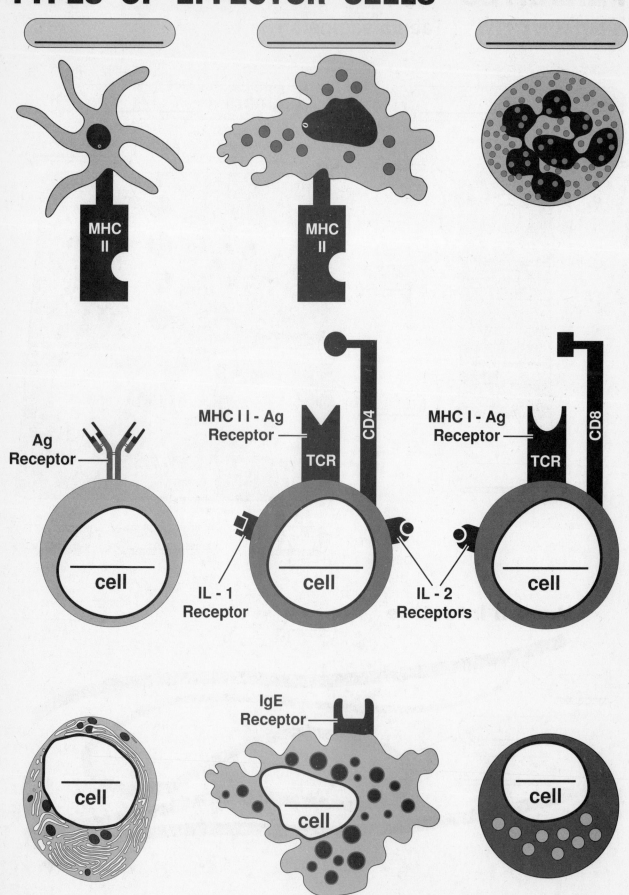

MACROPHAGES

Microbes ingested by macrophages stimulate the release of
_____ and _____

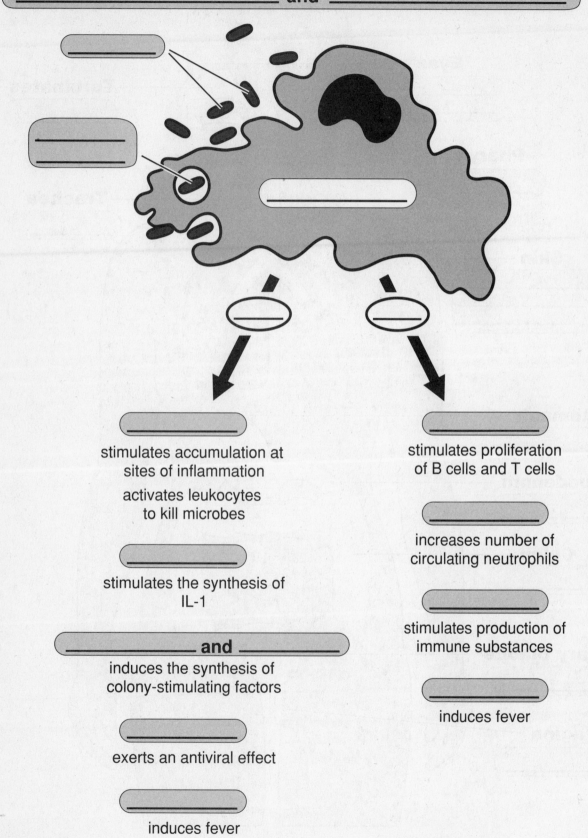

stimulates accumulation at
sites of inflammation

activates leukocytes
to kill microbes

stimulates the synthesis of
IL-1

_____ and _____

induces the synthesis of
colony-stimulating factors

exerts an antiviral effect

induces fever

stimulates proliferation
of B cells and T cells

increases number of
circulating neutrophils

stimulates production of
immune substances

induces fever

NONSPECIFIC BARRIERS TO INFECTION

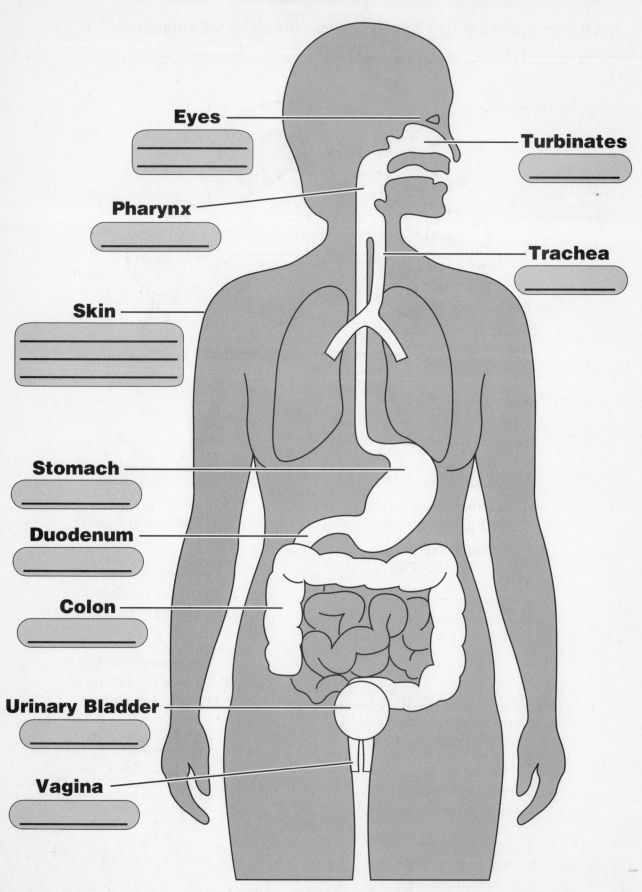

Eyes

Turbinates

Pharynx

Trachea

Skin

Stomach

Duodenum

Colon

Urinary Bladder

Vagina

INFLAMMATION

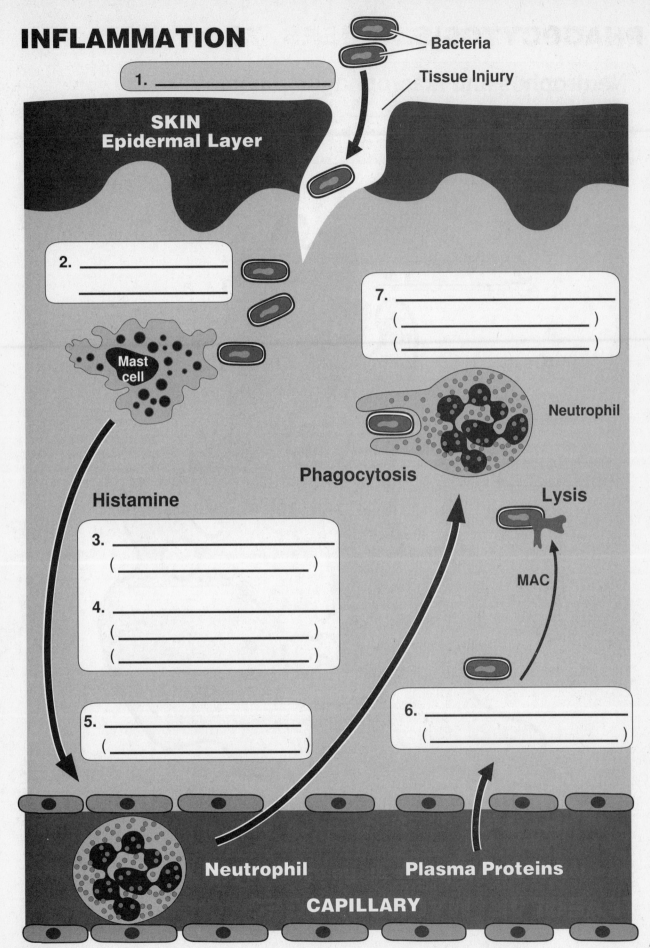

Bacteria

Tissue Injury

1. _____

SKIN
Epidermal Layer

2. _____
   _____

Mast cell

7. _____
   (_____)
   (_____)

Neutrophil

Phagocytosis

Lysis

Histamine

3. _____
   (_____)

4. _____
   (_____)
   (_____)

MAC

5. _____
   (_____)

6. _____
   (_____)

Neutrophil   **Plasma Proteins**

CAPILLARY

PHAGOCYTOSIS

Neutrophils and macrophages phagocytize
_____ , _____ , _____ ,
and foreign materials.

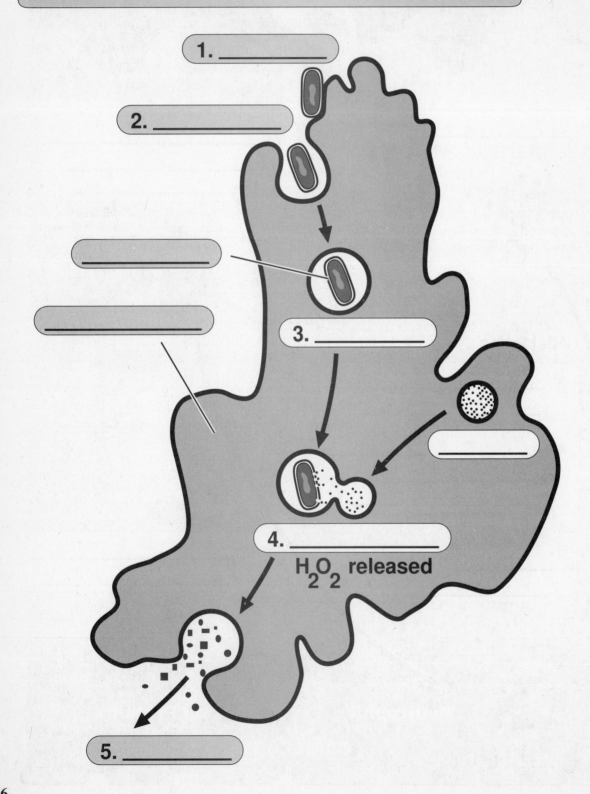

1. _____

2. _____

_____

_____

3. _____

_____

4. _____

H_2O_2 released

5. _____

MACROPHAGE LOCATIONS

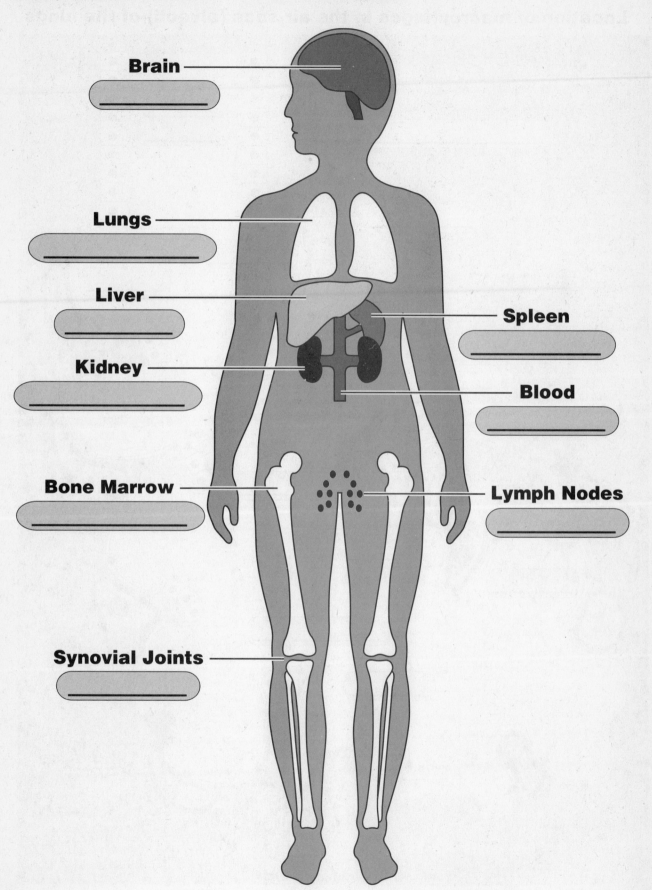

Brain

_____

Lungs

_____

Liver

_____

Spleen

_____

Kidney

_____

Blood

_____

Bone Marrow

_____

Lymph Nodes

_____

Synovial Joints

_____

ALVEOLAR MACROPHAGES
Location of macrophages in the air sacs (alveoli) of the lungs

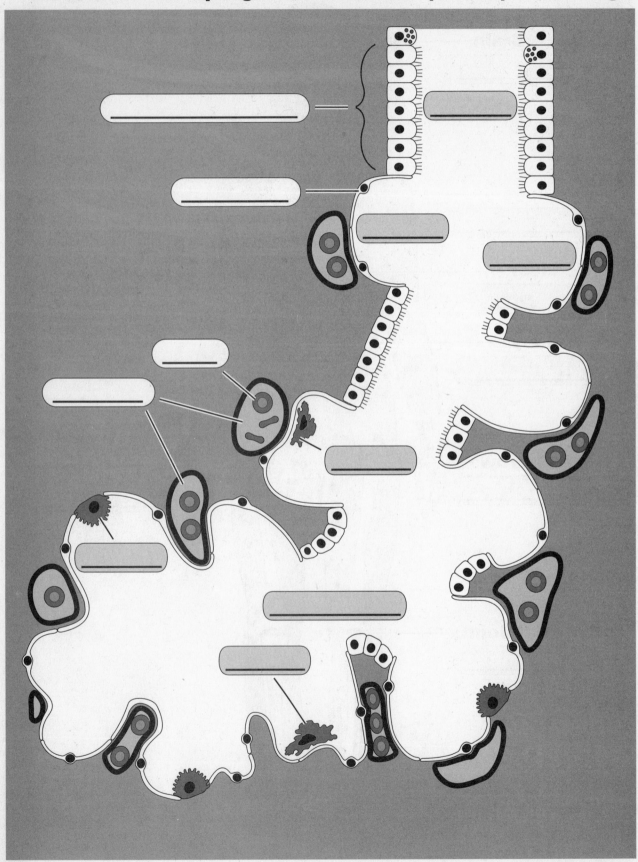

COMPLEMENT SYSTEM
Alternative Complement Pathway (nonspecific response)

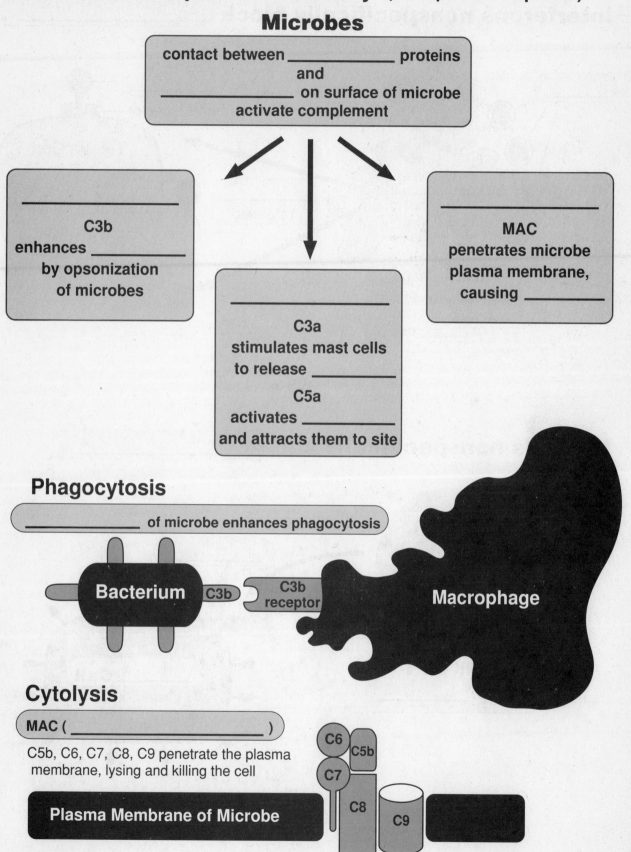

Microbes

contact between _____ proteins
and
_____ on surface of microbe
activate complement

_____
C3b
enhances _____
by opsonization
of microbes

_____
C3a
stimulates mast cells
to release _____
C5a
activates _____
and attracts them to site

_____
MAC
penetrates microbe
plasma membrane,
causing _____

Phagocytosis

_____ of microbe enhances phagocytosis

Bacterium C3b | C3b receptor | **Macrophage**

Cytolysis

MAC (_____)

C5b, C6, C7, C8, C9 penetrate the plasma
membrane, lysing and killing the cell

C6 C5b
C7
C8 C9

Plasma Membrane of Microbe

INTERFERONS AND NK CELLS

Interferons nonspecifically block [_____].

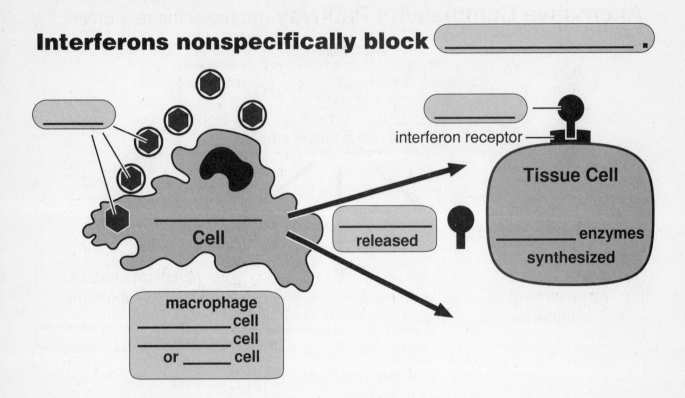

[_____]

interferon receptor

Tissue Cell

_____ enzymes synthesized

_____ Cell

[_____] released

macrophage
_____ cell
_____ cell
or _____ cell

NK cells nonspecifically kill [_____].

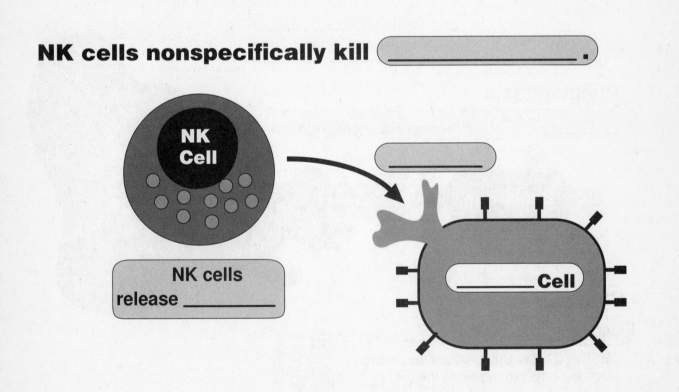

NK Cell

[_____]

NK cells release _____

_____ Cell

LYMPHATIC SYSTEM

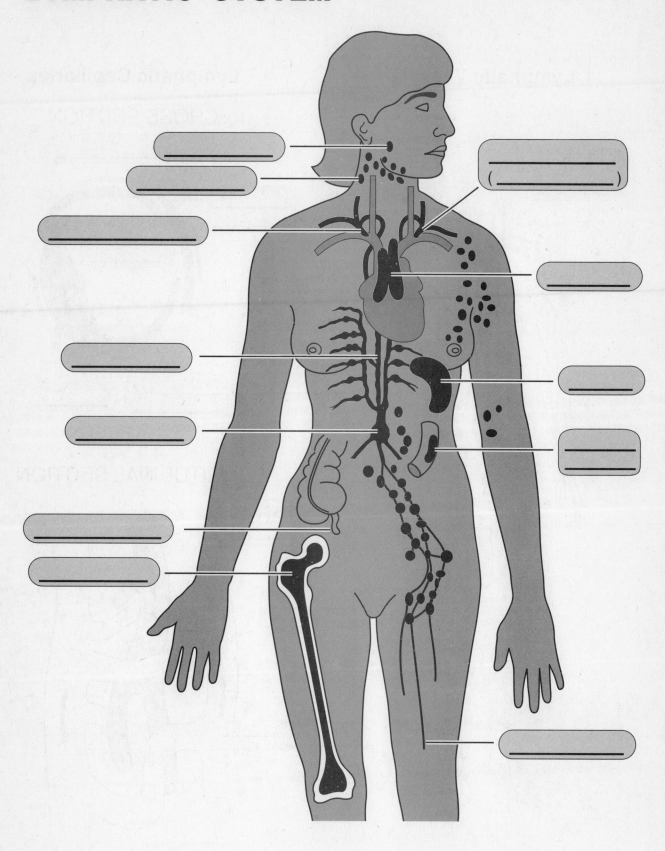

LYMPHATIC VESSELS

Lymphatic Vessels

Lymphatic Capillaries

CROSS SECTION

LONGITUDINAL SECTION

LYMPH TRUNKS AND LYMPHATIC DUCTS

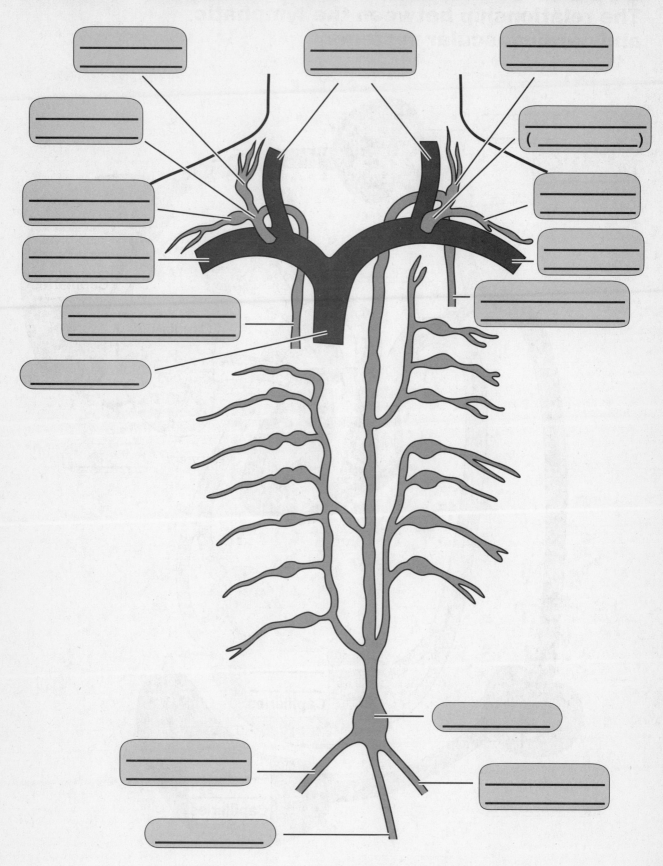

LYMPH AND BLOOD FLOW
The relationship between the lymphatic and cardiovascular systems

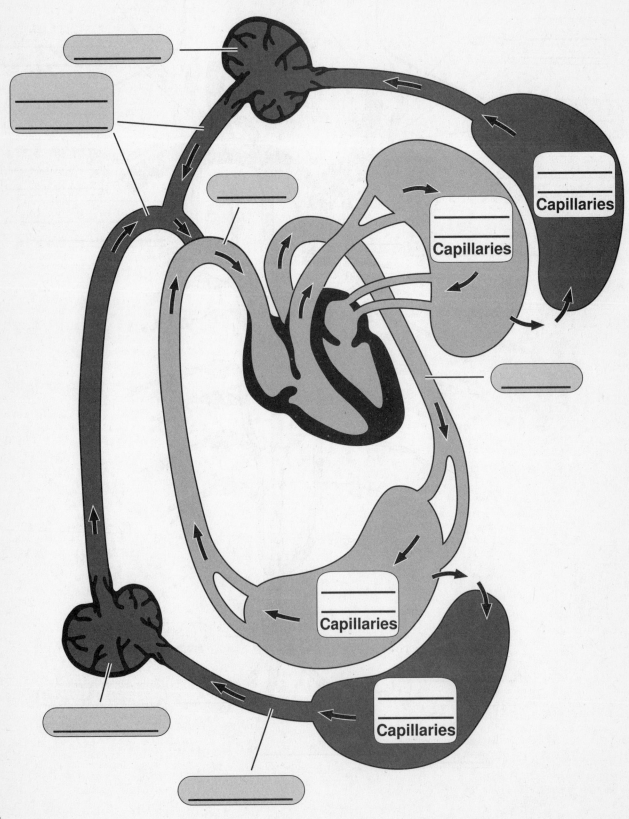

THYMUS GLAND

Immature T Cells : Immature T cells migrate from the _____ via the blood to the _____ , where they mature.

Mature T Cells : Mature T cells migrate from the thymus to specific regions in the _____ and the _____ , where they reside.

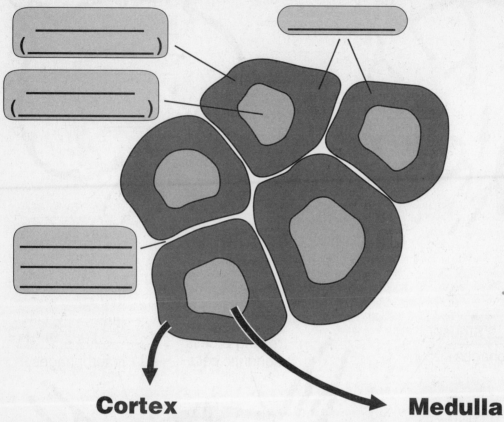

(_____)

(_____)

_____

Cortex

In the cortex of a lobule, reticular cells envelop groups of T cells that are multiplying and maturing.

Medulla

As T cells mature, they migrate to the medulla. Fully mature T cells leave the medulla via venules and efferent lymphatic vessels.

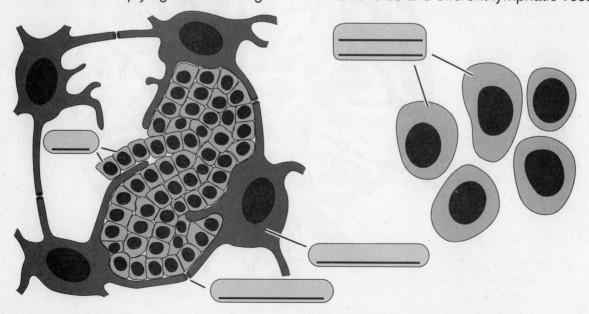

LYMPH NODE

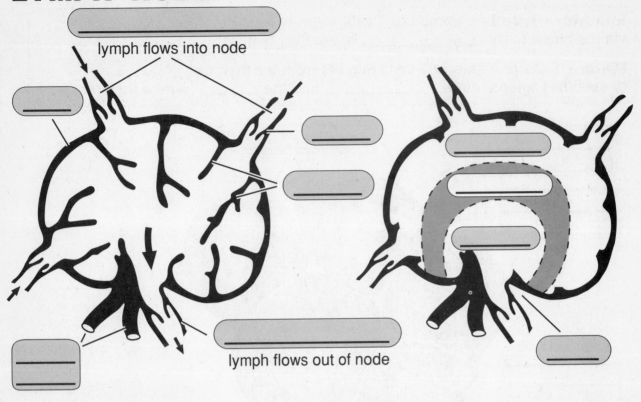

lymph flows into node

lymph flows out of node

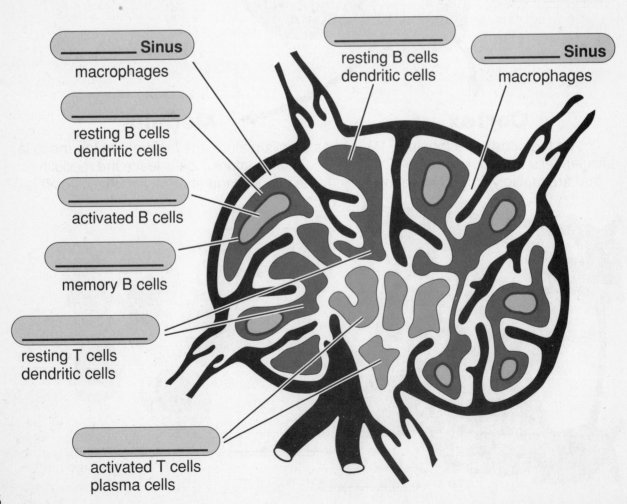

_____ **Sinus**
macrophages

resting B cells
dendritic cells

activated B cells

memory B cells

resting T cells
dendritic cells

_____

resting B cells
dendritic cells

_____ **Sinus**
macrophages

activated T cells
plasma cells

SPLEEN (schematic)

The spleen filters the blood. The main function of the spleen is the phagocytosis of bacteria and worn-out or damaged red blood cells.

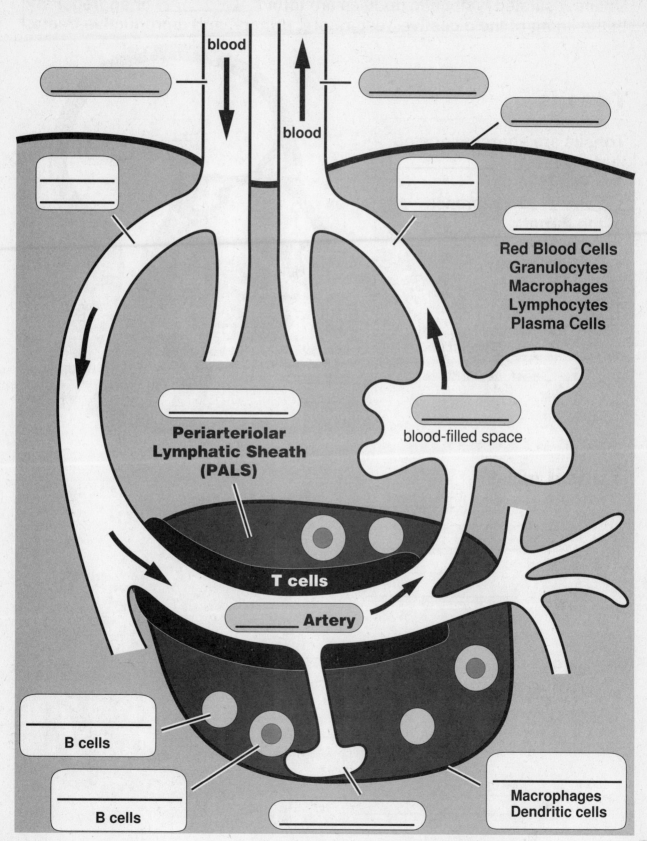

blood

blood

Red Blood Cells
Granulocytes
Macrophages
Lymphocytes
Plasma Cells

Periarteriolar Lymphatic Sheath (PALS)

blood-filled space

T cells

_____ Artery

B cells

B cells

Macrophages
Dendritic cells

DIFFUSE LYMPHATIC TISSUE

When lymphatic tissue is not enclosed by a capsule, it is called _____ or _____ lymphatic tissue.
Unencapsulated lymphatic nodules are found _____ or aggregated in the lining of the digestive, respiratory, urinary, and reproductive tracts.

Tonsils

Tonsils are aggregations of large lymphatic _____ embedded in the _____ membranes of the throat.

They form a ring of _____ tissue at the junction of the mouth cavity and _____ (throat).

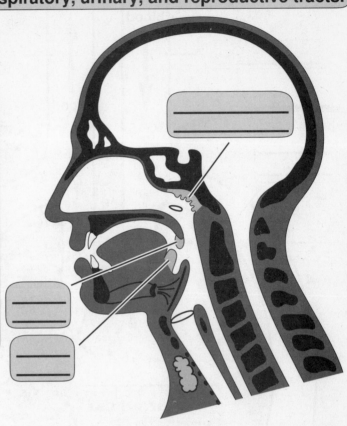

Tonsil (detail)

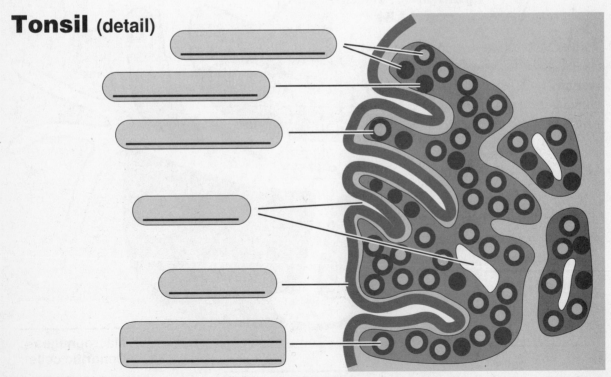

IMMUNIZATIONS
(Vaccinations against infectious diseases)

Disease	Comments
_____	Present in the Middle East and Asia; 2 injections (2 to 6 weeks apart); booster shots every 6 months
_____	Given in a series of 4 shots; booster shot every 7–10 years
_____	Recommended for all children 2 years old
_____	For people who do not test positive for antibodies to the hepatitis B virus and are at risk of acquiring the disease
_____	For the elderly and others at high risk of serious illness
_____	Should be given to children at age 15 months; inoculation is usually combined: measles-mumps-rubella
_____	Prevalent in regions of Africa and South America; types of vaccine : A, C, W-135, and Y
_____	Should be given to children at age 15 months; inoculation is usually combined: measles-mumps-rubella
_____ (_____)	Begun between 1 and 3 months of age; usually combined with tetanus and diptheria; should not be given to children over 6 years of age
_____	3 injections (one month or more apart)
_____	For elderly people before traveling; one dose only (3 weeks before departure); no further doses should be given
_____	Vaccine given orally at 2, 4, and 18 months of age; adults should also be immunized
_____	Common in domestic animals in India & South America; 3 injections at intervals of one week; booster injection 3 weeks later
_____	Should be given to children at age 15 months; inoculation is usually combined: measles-mumps-rubella
_____	Smallpox has been eradicated as of 1980; no vaccination is now needed.
_____	A series of shots completed by school age; a booster shot every 7 to 10 years for children over 12 and adults
_____	2 doses (at least one month apart); booster shot every 3 years

ANTIGENS

Antigens are molecules that are recognized as foreign .
Bacterial cells, virus-infected cells, cancer cells,
and the cells of disease-causing organisms
all have antigens that allow the body to recognize them as foreign.

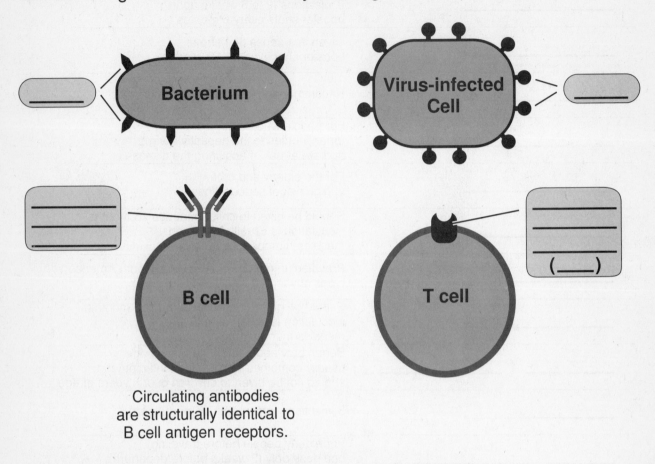

Bacterium

Virus-infected
Cell

B cell

T cell

Circulating antibodies
are structurally identical to
B cell antigen receptors.

(Epitopes)

A given antibody binds to a particular part of its antigen
called the antigenic determinant (or epitope).

Most antigen molecules have several different antigenic determinants.

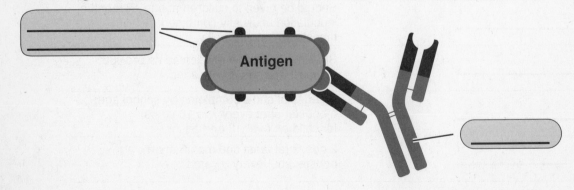

Antigen

ANTIBODY STRUCTURE
The Basic Antibody (Immunoglobulin) Structure

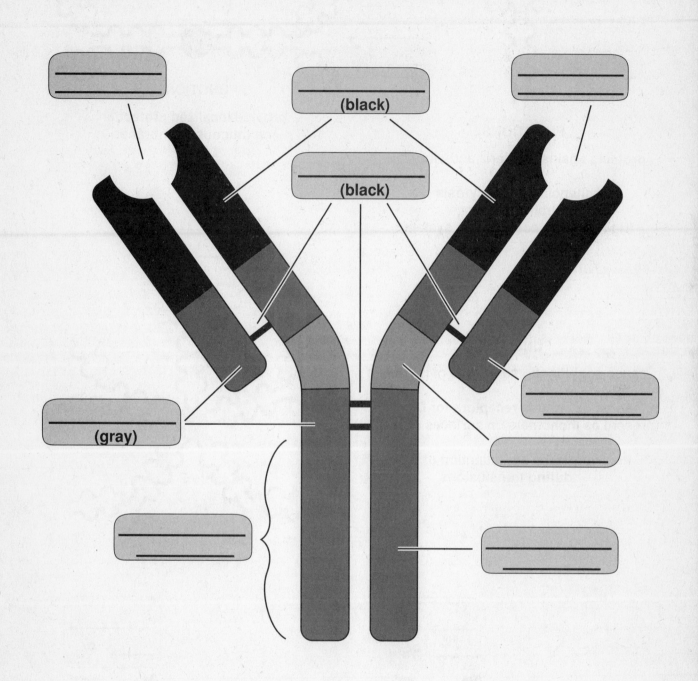

ANTIBODY CLASSIFICATION

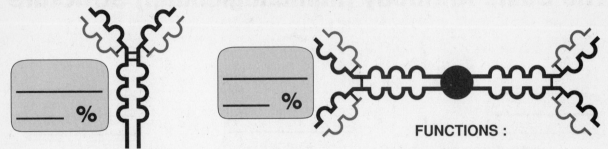

```
_____
____ %
```

FUNCTIONS :

protects against bacteria and viruses
by
enhancing phagocytosis
neutralizing toxins
triggering the complement system

```
_____
____ %
```

FUNCTIONS :

provide localized protection
on mucous membranes

FUNCTIONS :

cause agglutination and lysis of microbes

serve as antigen receptors for B cells
(present as monomers on surfaces of B cells)

involved in the agglutination of blood
during transfusions

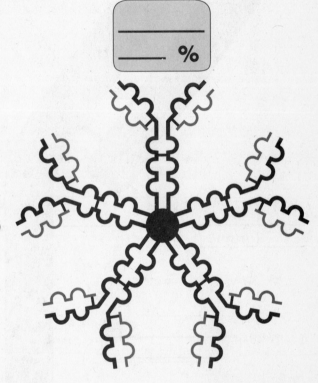

```
_____
____ %
```

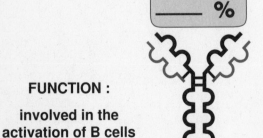

```
_____
____ %
```

FUNCTION :

involved in the
activation of B cells

```
_____
____ %
```

FUNCTION :

involved in the
allergic responses

LYMPHOCYTES
Origin, Maturation, and Locations in Lymphatic Tissues

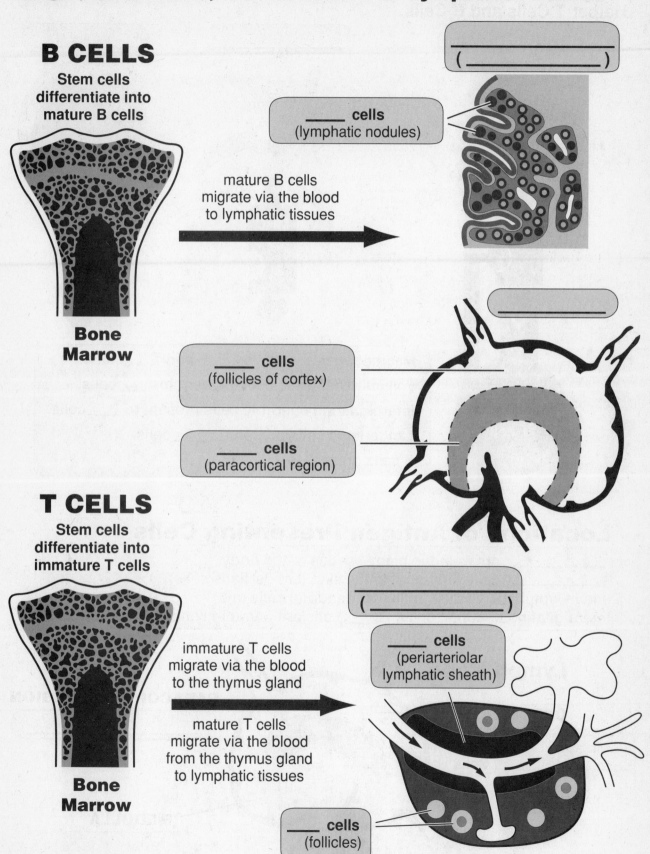

B CELLS
Stem cells differentiate into mature B cells

Bone Marrow

mature B cells migrate via the blood to lymphatic tissues

_____
(_____)

_____ cells (lymphatic nodules)

_____ cells (follicles of cortex)

_____ cells (paracortical region)

_____

T CELLS
Stem cells differentiate into immature T cells

Bone Marrow

immature T cells migrate via the blood to the thymus gland

mature T cells migrate via the blood from the thymus gland to lymphatic tissues

_____
(_____)

_____ cells (periarteriolar lymphatic sheath)

_____ cells (follicles)

ANTIGEN PRESENTING CELLS

Antigen Presenting Cells Process and Present Antigens to Helper T Cells and B Cells.

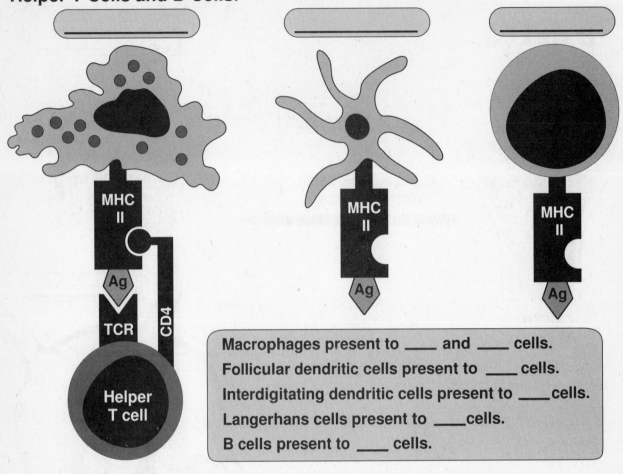

MHC II

Ag

TCR   CD4

Helper T cell

MHC II

Ag

MHC II

Ag

Macrophages present to ____ and ____ cells.
Follicular dendritic cells present to ____ cells.
Interdigitating dendritic cells present to ____ cells.
Langerhans cells present to ____ cells.
B cells present to ____ cells.

Locations of Antigen Presenting Cells

_____ are found in many tissues of the body.
_____ cells are found in the skin (Langerhans cells)
and in lymphatic tissues (follicular dendritic cells and
interdigitating dendritic cells). ____ cells are found in lymphatic tissues.

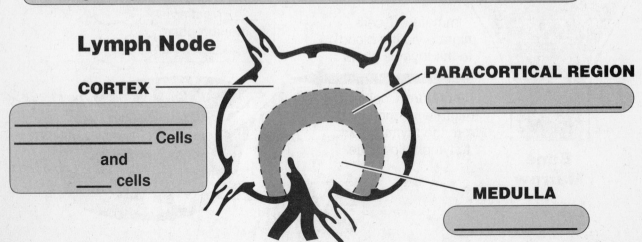

Lymph Node

CORTEX

PARACORTICAL REGION

_____ Cells
and
____ cells

MEDULLA

ANTIGEN PROCESSING
Example: A Macrophage Processing Bacterial Antigens

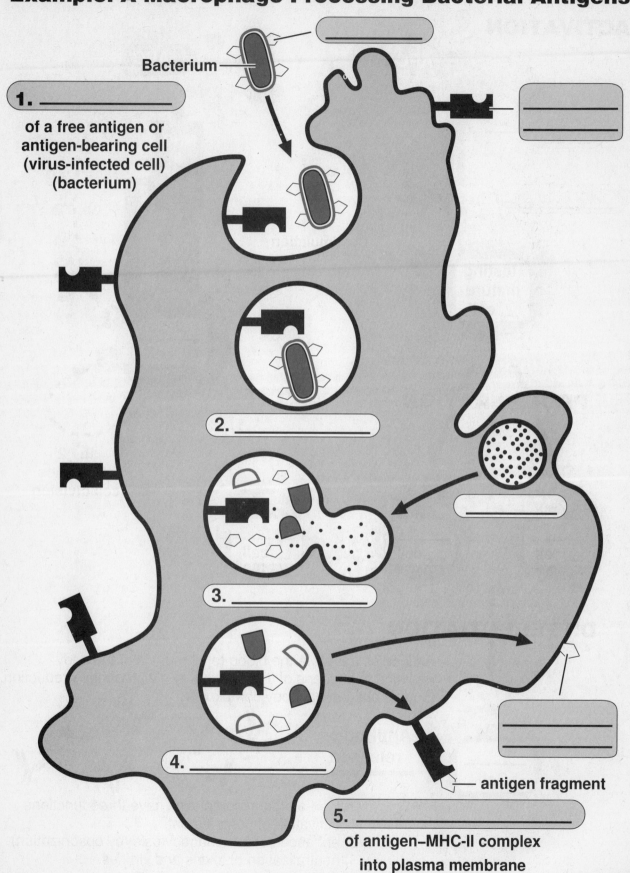

Bacterium

1. _____

of a free antigen or
antigen-bearing cell
(virus-infected cell)
(bacterium)

2. _____

3. _____

4. _____

5. _____

of antigen–MHC-II complex

into plasma membrane

antigen fragment

ANTIBODY–MEDIATED IMMUNITY

ACTIVATION

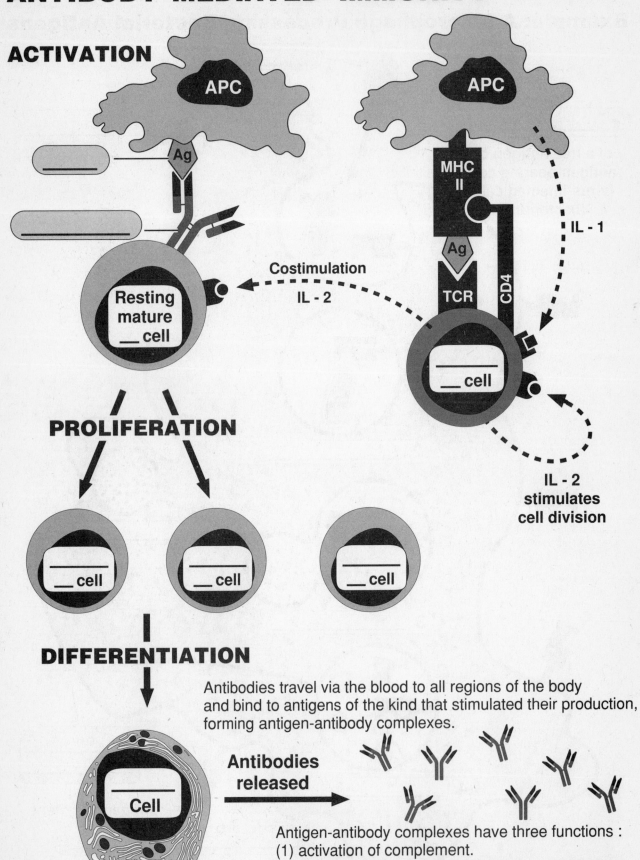

APC

APC

Ag

MHC II

Ag

IL - 1

Costimulation
IL - 2

TCR

CD4

Resting
mature
__ cell

__ cell

IL - 2
stimulates
cell division

PROLIFERATION

__ cell

__ cell

__ cell

DIFFERENTIATION

Antibodies travel via the blood to all regions of the body
and bind to antigens of the kind that stimulated their production,
forming antigen-antibody complexes.

**Antibodies
released**

Cell

Antigen-antibody complexes have three functions :
(1) activation of complement.
(2) enhancement of phagocytosis (by opsonization).
(3) neutralization of toxins and viruses.

ANTIBODY PRODUCTION IN LYMPH NODE

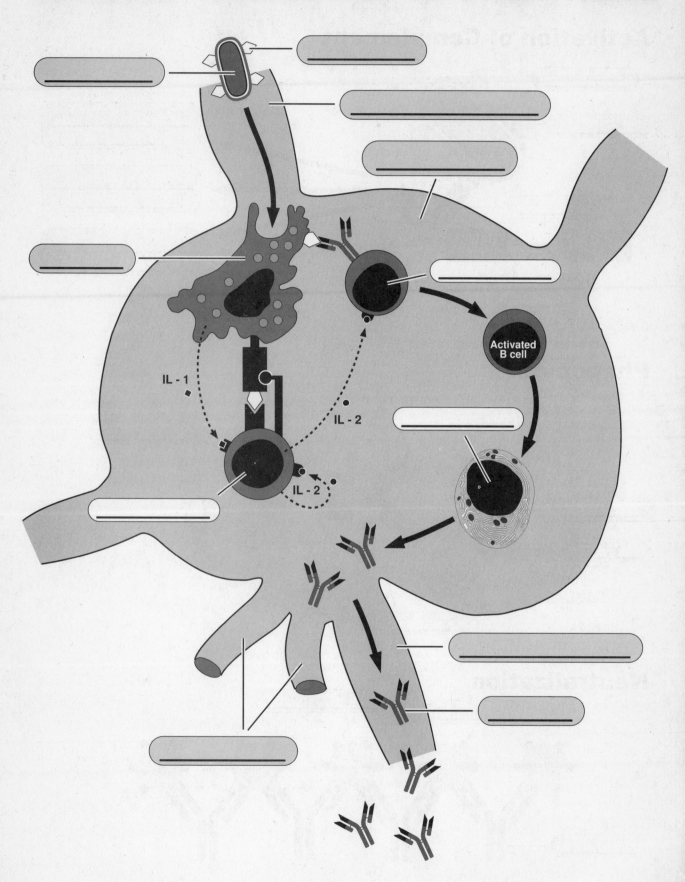

Activated
B cell

IL - 1

IL - 2

IL - 2

ANTIBODY FUNCTIONS

Activation of Complement

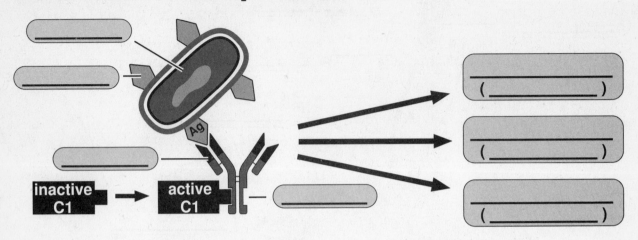

Phagocytosis

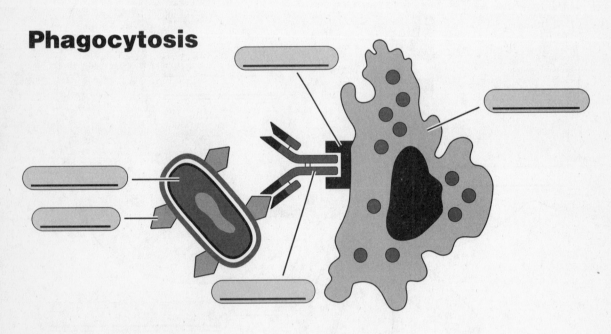

Neutralization

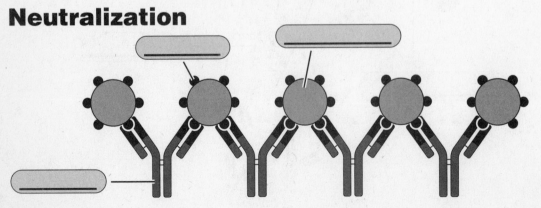

CELL–MEDIATED IMMUNITY

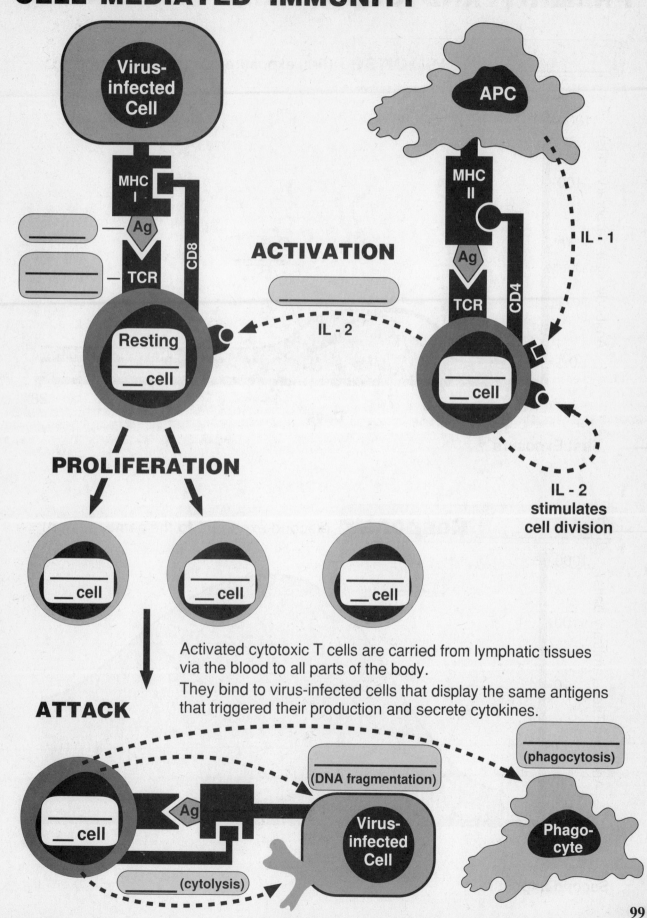

ACTIVATION

PROLIFERATION

Activated cytotoxic T cells are carried from lymphatic tissues via the blood to all parts of the body.

They bind to virus-infected cells that display the same antigens that triggered their production and secrete cytokines.

ATTACK

99

PRIMARY AND SECONDARY RESPONSES

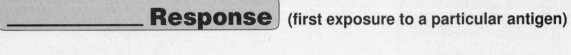

_____ **Response** (first exposure to a particular antigen)

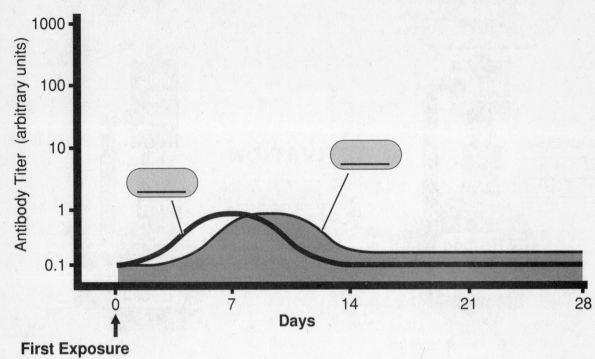

_____ **Response** (second exposure to the same antigen)

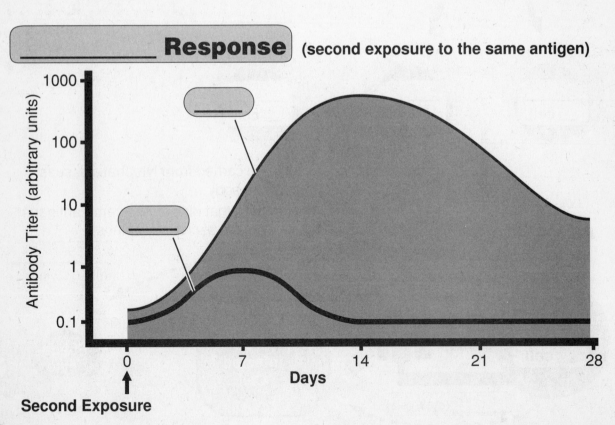

Part III : Terminology

Pronunciation Guide

adenoids   AD - e - noyds

adherence   ad - HĒR - ens

afferent   AF - er - ent

agglutination   a - glooˊ - ti - NĀ - shun

agglutinin   a - GLOO - ti - nin

agglutinogen   agˊ - loo - TIN - ō - jen

agranular   a - GRAN - yoo - lar

agranulocyte   a - GRAN - yoo - lō - sītˊ

allergen   AL - er - jen

allergic   a - LER - jik

alveolar   al - VĒ - ō - lar

alveolus   al - VĒ - ō - lus

anaphylaxis   anˊ - a - fi - LAK - sis

antibiotic   anˊ - ti - bī - OT - ik

antibody   AN - ti - bodˊ - ē

anticoagulant   anˊ - ti - kō - AG - yoo - lant

antigen   AN - ti - jen

antigenic   an - ti - JEN - ik

antimicrobial   anˊ - ti - mī - KRŌ - bē - al

anti-oncogene   anˊ - ti - ONG - kō - jēn

antiserum   anˊ - ti - SĒ - rum

antiviral   anˊ - ti - VĪ - ral

arteriole   ar - TĒ - rē - ōl

autocrine   AW - tō - krin

bacteria   bak - TĒ - rē - a

bactericidal   bak - tērˊ - i - SĪ - dal

bacterium   bak - TĒ - rē - um

basophil   BĀ - sō - fil

Billroth   BIL - rōt

bronchomediastinal   brongˊ - kō - mēˊ - dē - as - TĪ - nal

capillary   KAP - i - larˊ - ē

carcinogen   kar - SIN - ō - jen

carcinoma   karˊ - si - NŌ - ma

chemotactic   kēˊ - mō - TAK - tik

chemotaxis   kēˊ - mō - TAK - sis

cilia   SIL - ē - a

cilium   SIL - ē - um

cisterna chyli   sis - TER - na KĪ - lē

clone   KLŌN

commensal   ko - MEN - sal

cytokine   SĪ - tō - kīn

cytolysis   sī - TOL - i - sis

cytolytic   sīˊ - tō - LIT - ik

cytotoxic   sīˊ - tō - TOK - sik

defecation   def - e - KĀ - shun

dendritic   den - DRIT - ik

diapedesis   dīˊ - a - pe - DĒ - sis

disulfide   dī - SUL - fīd

efferent   EF - er - ent

endocytosis   enˊ - dō - sī - TŌ - sis

endogenous   en - DOJ - e - nus

endothelium   enˊ - dō - THĒ - lē - um

eosinophil   ēˊ - ō - SIN - ō - fil

epidermis   epˊ - i - DERM - is

epithelial   epˊ - i - THĒ - lē - al

epitope   EP - i - tōp

exogenous   eks - OJ - e - nus

fibrin   FĪ - brin

fibroblast   FĪ - brō - blast

follicle   **FOL - i - kul**
follicular   **fō - LIK - yoo - lar**
fungi   **FUN - jī**
fungus   **FUNG - gus**

granular   **GRAN - yoo - lar**
granulocyte   **GRAN - yoo - lō - sīt′**

hapten   **HAP - ten**
Hassall   **HAS - al**
hematopoiesis   **hem′ - a - tō - poy - Ē - sis**
hemopoiesis   **hē′ - mō - poy - Ē - sis**
hilus   **HĪ - lus**
histamine   **HISS - ta - mēn**
histocompatibility   **hiss′ - tō - kom - pat - i - BIL - i - tē**
humoral   **HYOO - mor - al**
hyaluronic   **hī′ - a - loo - RON - ik**
hybridoma   **hī′ - bri - DŌ - ma**
hydrolytic   **hī′ - drō - LIT - ik**

ileum   **IL - ē - um**
immunity   **im - YOO - ni - tē**
immunocompetence   **im′ - yoo - nō - KOM - pe - tens**
immunogen   **IM - yoo - nō - jen**
immunogenicity   **im′ - yoo - nō - je - NIS - i - tē**
immunoglobulin   **im′ - yoo - nō - GLOB - yoo - lin**
immunological   **im′ - yoo - nō - LOJ - i - kal**
immunology   **im′ - yoo - NOL - ō - jē**
immunosuppression   **im′ - yoo - nō - su - PRESH - un**
immunotherapy   **im′ - yoo - nō - THER - a - pē**
infection   **in - FEK - shun**
infectious   **in - FEK - shus**
interdigitating   **in′ - ter - DIJ - i - tā - ting**
interferon   **in′ - ter - FĒR - on**
interleukin   **in′ - ter - LOO - kin**
interstitial   **in′ - ter - STISH - al**
intestinal   **in - TES - ti - nal**

jugular   **JUG - yoo - lar**

keratinized   **KER - a - tin - izd**
kinin   **KĪ - nin**
Kupffer   **KOOP - fer**

lacrimal   **LAK - ri - mal**
lamina propria   **LAM - i - na PRŌ - prē - a**
Langerhans   **LANG - er - hanz**
leukemia   **loo - KĒ - mē - a**
leukocyte   **LOO - kō - sīt**
leukocytosis   **loo′ - kō - sī - TŌ - sis**
leukopenia   **loo′ - kō - PĒ - nē - a**
leukotriene   **loo′ - kō - TRĪ - ēn**
lingual   **LIN - gwal**
lobule   **LOB - yool**

lumbar   **LUM - bar**
lumen   **LOO - men**
lymph   **LYMF**
lymphatic   **lim - FAT - ik**
lymphocyte   **LIM - fō - sīt**
lymphokine   **LIM - fō - kīn**
lymphotoxin   **lim′ - fō - TOK - sin**
lysis   **LĪ - sis**
lysosome   **LĪ - sō - sōm**
lysozyme   **LĪ - sō - zīm**

macrophage   **MAK - rō - fāj**
margination   **mar′ - ji - NĀ - shun**
mediator   **MĒ - dē - ā - tor**
medulla   **me - DULL - la**
medullary   **MED - yoo - lar′ - ē**
microbe   **MĪ - krōb**
microglia   **mī - KROG - lē - a**
microorganism   **mī′ - krō - OR - gan - izm**
microphage   **MĪK - rō - fāj**
mitosis   **mī - TŌ - sis**
mitotic   **mī - TOT - ik**
molecule   **MOL - e - kyool**
monoclonal   **mon′ - ō - KLŌN - al**
monocyte   **MON - ō - sīt**
monokine   **MON - ō - kīn**
mononuclear   **mon′ - ō - NOO - klē - ar**
mucosa   **myoo - KŌ - sa**
mucous   **MYOO - kus**
mucus   **MYOO - kus**
mutation   **myoo - TĀ - shun**

necrosis   **ne - KRŌ - sis**
neutrophil   **NOO - trō - fil**
nodule   **NOD - yool**
nucleus   **NOO - klē - us**

oncogene   **ONG - kō - jēn**
oncology   **ong - KOL - ō - jē**
opsonin   **OP - sō - nin**
opsonization   **op′ - sō - ni - ZĀ - shun**
oxidant   **OK - si - dant**

palatine   **PAL - a - tīn**
paracortical   **par′ - a - KOR - ti - kal**
paracrine   **PAR - a - krin**
pathogen   **PATH - ō - jen**
pathogenesis   **path′ - ō - JEN - e - sis**
pathological   **path′ - ō - LOJ - i - kal**
perforin   **PER - fō - rin**
periarteriolar   **per′ - ē - ar - TĒR - ē - ō - lar**
Peyer   **PĪ - er**
phagocyte   **FAG - ō - sīt**
phagocytic   **fag′ - ō - SIT - ik**

phagocytosis fag′-ō-sī-TŌ-sis
phagolysosome fag′-ō-LĪ-sō-sōm
phagosome FAG-ō-sōm
pharyngeal fa-RIN-jē-al
pharynx FAR-inks
pluripotent ploo-RIP-ō-tent
pneumonia noo-MŌ-nē-a
progeny PROJ-e-nē
proliferation pro-lif′-er-Ā-shun
properdin prō-PER-din
prostaglandin pros′-ta-GLAN-din
proto-oncogene prō′-tō-ONG-kō-jēn
protozoa prō′-tō-ZŌ-a
pus PUS

replication rep′-li-KĀ-shun
residual re-ZID-yoo-al
resistance re-ZIS-tans
respiratory RES-pi-ra-tor-ē
reticular re-TIK-yoo-lar
reticuloendothelial re-tik′-yoo-lō-en′-dō-THĒ-lē-al
retrovirus ret′-rō-VĪ-rus

saliva sa-LĪ-va
salivary SAL-i-ver-ē
sebaceous se-BĀ-shus
sebum SĒ-bum
secretion se-KRĒ-shun
serum SĒ-rum
sinus SĪ-nus
sinusoid SĪN-yoo-soyd
specificity spes′-i-FIS-i-tē
spleen SPLĒN
splenic SPLĒN-ik
stellate STEL-āt
subclavian sub-KLĀ-vē-an
sudoriferous soo′-dor-IF-er-us
surveillance sur-VĀL-ans

thoracic thō-RAS-ik
titer TĪ-ter
tonsil TON-sil
toxic TOK-sik
toxoid TOK-soyd
trabecula tra-BEK-yoo-la
trabeculae tra-BEK-yoo-lē
transcriptase trans-KRIP-tās
transferrin trans-FER-rin
transfusion trans-FYOO-zhun
tubercle bacillus TOO-ber-kul ba-SIL-us

vaginal VAJ-i-nal
vasoconstriction vas′-ō-kon-STRIK-shun
vasodilation vas′-ō-dī-LĀ-shun

venous sinus VĒ-nus SĪ-nus
venule VEN-yool
vermiform appendix VER-mi-form a-PEN-diks
vesicle VES-i-kul

Glossary of Terms

Acquired immune deficiency syndrome (AIDS)   A disorder characterized by a positive HIV-antibody test and certain indicator diseases (Kaposi's sarcoma, *Pneumocystis carinii* pneumonia, tuberculosis, fungus diseases, etc.), a deficiency of helper T cells that results in fever or night sweats, coughing, sore throat, fatigue, body aches, weight loss, and enlarged lymph nodes.   Caused by a virus called human immunodeficiency virus (HIV).

Adenoids   The pharyngeal tonsil.

Adherence   The attachment of the plasma membrane of a phagocyte to the surface of a microbe or other foreign substance.   Adherence to some microbes is difficult; such microbes require opsonization (coating of the microbe with antibodies or C3b complement fragments).   Receptors on the surface of the phagocyte bind with antibodies or C3b fragments on the surface of the microbe.

Afferent   To carry toward.   In the lymphatic system, the term applies to lymphatic vessels that carry lymph into lymph nodes.

Agglutination   Clumping of microbes or red blood cells; typically an antigen-antibody reaction.

Agglutinin   An antibody in blood serum that is capable of causing red blood cells to clump.   Also called *isoantibody*.

Agglutinogen   An antigen located on the surface of red blood cells.   Agglutinogens are the basis for the ABO grouping and Rh system of blood classification.   Also called an *isoantigen*.

Aggregated lymphatic follicles   Aggregations (clusters) of lymphatic nodules that are found in the mucous membrane lining the gastrointestinal tract.   Examples include the tonsils (in the throat), Peyer's patches (in the small intestine), and the appendix (attached to the cecum of the ascending colon).

Agranular leukocyte   A white blood cell that does not have granules.   Includes lymphocytes and monocytes.   Also called *agranulocyte*.

Agranulocyte   *See* Agranular leukocyte.

AIDS   *See* Acquired immune deficiency syndrome.

Allergen   An antigen that evokes an allergic (hypersensitive) reaction.

Allergic   Pertaining to or sensitive to an allergen.   Also called *hypersensitive*.

Allergy   A secondary immune response to an antigen, resulting in tissue damage.   Also called *hypersensitivity*.

Alternative complement pathway   A sequence of complement activation that is not antibody-dependent.   It is triggered by the binding of one of the complement proteins (C3) to certain sugar molecules on the surface of a microbe.   Activated complement enhances inflammation, kills microbes by cytolysis, and enhances phagocytosis (by coating microbes with C3b).

Alveolar macrophage   A macrophage (phagocytic cell) found in the air sacs (alveoli) of the lungs.   Also called a *dust cell*.

Anaphylaxis   An immediate allergic reaction following the introduction of an antigen into a sensitized (primed) individual.   IgE antibodies attach to mast cells and basophils, causing them to produce mediators of anaphylaxis (hista-mine, leukotrienes, kinins, and prostaglandins) that bring about increased permeability of blood vessels, increased smooth muscle contraction, and increased mucus production.   Examples are hay fever, hives, and anaphylactic shock.   Also called *type I hypersensitivity*.

Antibiotic   Literally, "anti-life"; a chemical produced by a microorganism that is able to kill or inhibit the growth of other microorganisms.

Antibody (Ab)   A protein produced by plasma cells.   When activated by an antigen, B cells differentiate into plasma cells.   The antibodies produced by a particular plasma cell combine with the same type of antigen that stimulated their production, forming antigen-antibody complexes.   Also called *immunoglobulin* or *Ig*.

Antibody-mediated immunity (AMI)   A specific response to infection.   B cells activated by antigens develop into plasma cells that produce antibodies.   AMI is the immune response used to attack microbes and foreign substances present in the body fluids; especially bacteria.   Also called *humoral immunity*.

Antibody titer   A measure of the concentration of antibodies.

Anticoagulant   A substance that is able to delay, suppress, or prevent the clotting of blood.

Antigen (Ag)   Any substance that when introduced into the tissues or blood elicits a specific immune response (the activation of B cells or T cells).   Previously an antigen was defined as a substance that induces the production of antibodies (*anti* = antibodies; *gen* = generates.)

Antigen-binding site   The region of an antibody that binds specifically to an antigenic determinant.   Most antibodies have two antigen-binding sites, one at the tip of each variable region.

Antigenic determinant   The specific portion of an antigen that triggers an immune response.   T cell antigen receptors (TCRs) and antibodies bind to antigenic determinants.   The number of different antigenic determinants in the environment is enormous, and each type of antigenic determinant can elicit the formation of specific antibodies or T cells that are directed against it.   Also called an *epitope*.

Antigen-presenting cell (APC)   A cell that processes and presents antigens to B cells or T cells.   The three types of antigen-presenting cells are macrophages, dendritic cells, and some B cells.

Antigen receptor   A protein molecule located on the surface of a B cell or T cell that binds to a specific antigen (antigenic determinant).   B cell antigen receptors have the same chemical structure as the antibodies they will ultimately produce.   T cell antigen receptor is abbreviated TCR.

Antimicrobial substances   Chemicals that are involved in killing or inhibiting the growth of microbes.   They provide a second line of defense should microbes penetrate the skin or mucous membranes.   Examples include complement proteins, interferens, transferrins, and properdin.

Anti-oncogene   A gene that may produce proteins that normally oppose the action of an oncogene (cancer-producing gene) or inhibit cell division.   Mutation of an anti-oncogene is the most common genetic change in a wide variety of cancer cells.

Antiserum   A serum (blood plasma minus clotting factors) containing induced antibodies.

Appendix   *See* Vermiform appendix.

Arteriole   A small, almost microscopic, artery that delivers blood to a capillary.

Athlete's foot   A fungus infection that develops on the surface of the skin when the environment is warm and moist.

Autocrine   Local hormone that acts on the same cell that secreted it. An example is interleukin-2 (IL-2); it is secreted by activated helper T cells, and it stimulates the same helper T cells to proliferate.

Autoimmune diseases   Disorders that result from an immunological response against a person's own tissue antigens.

Bacteria (singular : bacterium)   All prokaryotic organisms, except the blue-green algae. Prokaryotic organisms are single-celled organisms that do not contain a membrane-bound nucleus. (*pro* = before; *karyon* = nucleus)

Bactericidal substance   A substance that is destructive to bacteria.

Basement membrane   A layer of extracellular material that attaches epithelial tissue to the underlying connective tissue; consists of the basal lamina and reticular lamina.

Basophil   A type of white blood cell characterized by large granules that stain with basic dyes. Basophils enter tissues and become mast cells, which secrete histamine. Basophils increase during allergic reactions.

B cell   A lymphocyte that develops into antibody-secreting plasma cells when activated by a specific antigen. Its functions include defense against bacteria, viruses in the extracellular fluid, and toxins. It can also function as an antigen presenting cell for helper T cells. Also called a *B lymphocyte*.

Billroth's cords   *See* Splenic cords.

B lymphocyte   *See* B cell.

Body cavity   A space within the body that contains various internal organs.

Bone marrow   The site of production of white blood cells and red blood cells.

Cancer   A malignant tumor that originates in epithelial cells. It tends to infiltrate and give rise to new growths. Also called *carcinoma*.

Capillary   A microscopic blood vessel located between an arteriole and venule through which materials are exchanged between blood and body cells.

Carcinogen   Any substance that causes cancer.

Carcinoma   *See* Cancer.

Carrier molecule   A large molecule to which a hapten (partial antigen) can bind; as a result, the hapten is rendered immunogenic (capable of triggering an immune response).

Cell-mediated immunity (CMI)   A specific response to infection mediated by T cells. T cells activated by antigens bind to cells that display the same antigens and kill them by cytolysis. CMI is the immune response used to kill cancer cells and virus-infected cells. Also called *cellular immunity*.

Chemical mediators   Chemicals that play important roles in the defense mechanisms of the body. They include plasma proteins (such as complement proteins, antibodies, kinins, and clotting factors) and cytokines, which are chemicals secreted by lymphocytes, macrophages, or monocytes.

Chemotactic agents   Chemicals that attract phagocytes to a site of infection or tissue damage. They include certain complement proteins and substances released from damaged tissue cells, white blood cells, and microbes.

Chemotaxis   Attraction of phagocytes to microbes or damaged tissue by a chemical stimulus.

Cilium (plural : cilia)   A hairlike process projecting from a cell that may be used to move the entire cell or to move substances along the surface of the cell. Cilia lining the trachea sweep mucus upward; when it reaches the opening to the esophagus, the mucus is swallowed.

Cisterna chyli   The dilated first portion of the thoracic duct; it receives lymph from the intestinal trunk and the right and left lumbar trunks. It is located in front of the second lumbar vertebra.

Classical complement pathway   A sequence of complement activation that is antibody-dependent. It is triggered by the binding of one of the complement proteins (C1) to an antibody-antigen complex. Activated complement enhances inflammation, kills microbes by cytolysis, and enhances phagocytosis (by coating microbes with C3b).

Clone   A population of identical cells. The descendents of a single cell that have been produced asexually (by mitosis).

Colony-stimulating factor (CSF)   One of a group of cytokines that stimulates development of white blood cells. Examples are macrophage CSF and granulocyte CSF.

Commensal bacteria   If a close and permanent association between organisms of different species benefits one species and neither benefits nor harms the other species, it is called commensalism. Certain pathogenic bacteria live on the moist secretions of mucous membranes; if present in sufficient numbers, they may be able to invade the membrane.

Complement system   A group of at least 20 normally inactive proteins found in blood plasma. When activated, they participate in specific (immune) and nonspecific responses to infection. The classical pathway is triggered by the binding of C1 to an antigen-antibody complex. The alternative pathway is triggered by the binding of C3 to polysaccharides on the surface of a microbe. Activated complement proteins enhance the inflammatory response, kill microbes directly by cytolysis, and enhance phagocytosis.

Connective tissue   The most abundant of the four basic tissue types of the body. It binds together, supports, and strengthens other tissues; protects and insulates internal organs; and compartmentalizes structures such as skeletal muscles.

Cortex   The outer layer of an organ. In the lymphatic system, the thymus gland and lymph nodes have a cortex.

Costimulator   A *second signal* that is needed for a B cell or T cell to become activated. Antigen recognition (binding) by an antigen receptor is the *first signal* required for B or T cell activation. Examples of costimulators are interleukin-1 (secreted by macrophages) and interleukin-2 (secreted by activated helper T cells).

Cytokines   Substances produced by activated lymphocytes and other cells. Cytokines act as autocrines or paracrines; they have a variety of roles in immunity and blood cell development. Monokines (secreted by monocytes and macrophages) and lymphokines (secreted by lymphocytes) are collectively referred to as cytokines.

Cytolysis   Killing of target cells by membrane lysis. the cytokine perforin, secreted by activated cytotoxic T cells, forms holes in the cell membrane of the target cell, causing it to burst and die. A group of complement proteins called the membrane attack complex (MAC) penetrate the plasma membrane of the target cell, lysing and killing it. Also called *lysis*.

Cytotoxic Cells or antibodies that damage target cells.

Cytotoxic T cell (Tc cell) T lymphocyte that, when activated, directly attacks virus-infected cells and tumor cells that display the same type of antigen that stimulated its activation. Bind antigen associated with MHC class I proteins. Also called a *cytolytic T cell*.

Defecation The discharge of feces from the rectum. Microbes that irritate the lining of the GI tract cause vigorous muscular contractions that result in diarrhea and rapid expulsion of microbes.

Delayed type hypersensitivity (DTH) An allergic response mediated by T cells. It is called delayed hypersensitivity because it takes several days to develop. An example is the skin rash caused by poison ivy. Also called a *cell-mediated hypersensitivity reaction* or *type IV hypersensitivity reaction.*.

Dendritic cells Antigen presenting cells that have long, branchlike projections. They are not phagocytic and express antigen associated with MHC II proteins. They are strategically located where antigens are likely to penetrate nonspecific defenses and enter the body, especially in the mucous membranes and the skin.

Diapedesis The passage of white blood cells through the walls of blood capillaries. The white blood cells squeeze through the spaces (intercellular clefts) between the endothelial cells that comprise the capillary walls. Also called *emigration*.

Differentiation Acquisition of specific functions different from those of the original cell.

Diffuse lymphatic tissue Lymphatic tissue that is not enclosed by a capsule. It is found in small amounts in almost every organ of the body. Specific examples include the tonsils and aggregated lymphatic nodules of the intestinal mucosa (Peyer's patches). Also called *unencapsulated lymphatic tissue*.

Edema An abnormal accumulation of interstitial fluid. During inflammation, it results from increased permeability of blood capillaries, which permits more plasma to filter into the tissue spaces.

Effector cell A cell involved in an immune response.

Efferent To carry away. In the lymphatic system, the term applies to lymphatic vessels that carry lymph away from lymph nodes.

Emigration *See* Diapedesis.

Endocytosis The uptake of materials by cells. Includes the uptake of water by pinocytosis and the uptake of large particles and cells by phagocytosis. In pinocytosis the plasma membrane folds into the cell, forming small intracellular vesicles filled with extracellular fluid; in phagocytosis, extensions of the plasma membrane (pseudopodia) surround the particle or cell and fuse, forming an intracellular vesicle.

Endogenous Growing from or beginning within the organism. For example, the antigens that appear on the surfaces of virus-infected cells are called endogenous antigens.

Endothelium The layer of simple squamous epithelial cells that lines the blood vessels, lymphatic vessels, and heart.

Eosinophil A type of white blood cell characterized by granules that stain with eosin dye. It is involved allergic responses and the destruction of parasitic worms.

Epidermis The outermost layer of the skin, composed of stratified squamous epithelium. It consists of many layers of closely packed cells called keratinocytes. Keratinocytes produce the protein keratin that helps waterproof and protect the skin and underlying tissues. Anchoring junctions called desmosomes weld keratinocytes to one another. The epidermis provides a physical barrier to the entrance of microbes. Periodic shedding of epidermal cells helps remove microbes on the skin surface. When the epithelal surface is broken, staphylococci, which normally inhabit hair follicles and sudoriferous (sweat) glands, are the most likely bacteria to enter the tissues and cause infection.

Epithelial tissue The tissue that forms glands or the outer part of the skin and lines blood vessels, hollow organs, and passages that lead externally from the body.

Epitope *See* Antigenic determinant.

Exocytosis A process of discharging celluluar products too large to go through the plasma membrane of a cell. An intracellular vesicle fuses with the plasma membrane, opens, and releases its contents into the extracellular fluid.

Exogenous Originating outside the body. For example, the antigens displayed on the surfaces of bacteria are called exogenous antigens.

Extracellular fluid (ECF) Fluid outside body cells. Interstitial fluid, blood plasma, and lymph.

Fever An elevation in body temperature above its normal level of 37 degrees centigrade (98.6 degrees Fahrenheit). It inhibits the growth of some microbes, intensifies the effects of interferons, and speeds up tissue repair processes.

Fibrin An insoluble protein that is essential to blood clotting. It is formed from fibrinogen by the action of thrombin.

Fibroblast A large, flat cell that forms collagen, elastic fibers, and the intercellular substance of areolar connective tissue. Secretes cytokines.

Filtration The passage of a liquid through a filter or membrane that acts as a filter. For example, the passage of blood plasma through the wall of a capillary into the spaces between the tissues cells, forming interstitial fluid.

Fixed macrophage Stationary phagocytic cell found in the liver, lungs, brain, spleen, lymph nodes, skin (subcutaneous tissue), and bone marrow. Also called a *histiocyte*.

Follicle Spherical region of densely packed lymphocytes, especially B cells. Follicles are found in lymph nodes, spleen, and diffuse lymphatic tissue. Also called *lymphatic nodules*.

Fungus (plural: fungi) A group of plantlike organisms, including mushrooms, yeasts, molds, rusts, etc. They cannot be classified as plants because they contain no chlorophyll (inability to make their own food by photosynthesis). Examples of infections caused by fungi include vaginal yeast infection, athlete's foot, thrush, ringworm, diaper rash, and jock itch.

Germinal center The central region of an active lymphatic nodule; contains activated B cells dividing and differentiating into plasma cells. The nodules are found in lymph nodes, the spleen, or diffuse lymphatic tissue.

Granular leukocyte   A white blood cell that contains cytoplasmic granules. There are three types: neutrophils, eosinophils, and basophils. Neutrophils and eosinophils are phagocytic granulocytes; basophils enter tissues and become mast cells, which secrete histamine and heparin. Also called *granulocyte*.

Granulocyte   *See* Granular leukocyte.

Hapten   A small molecule that is not immunogenic by itself. When coupled to a carrier molecule, it can elicit the production of antibodies directed against itself. An example is the small lipid toxin in poison ivy that triggers an immune response after combining with a body protein. Also called a *partial antigen*.

Hair follicle   Epithelium surrounding the root of a hair from which hair develops.

Helper T cell (T$_H$ cell)   A class of T cell that participates in both cell-mediated and antibody-mediated immune responses. It secretes cytokines that participate in the costimulation of cytotoxic T cells and B cells. It binds antigens associated with MHC class II proteins.

Hemopoiesis   Blood cell production occurring in the red marrow of bones. Also called *hematopoiesis*.

Hilus   An area, depression, or pit where blood vessels and nerves enter or leave an organ. Also called a *hilum*.

Histamine   Substance found in many cells, especially mast cells, basophils, and platelets. Released when the cells are injured. Causes vasodilation, increased permeability of blood vessels, and bronchiole constriction.

Histocompatibility testing   Comparison of human leukocyte associated antigens (HLAs) between donor and recipient to determine histocompatibility, the degree of compatibility between the two. Also called *HLA antigen typing* or *tissue typing*.

Hives   Condition of the skin marked by reddened elevated patches that are often itchy; may be caused by infections, trauma, medications, emotional stess, food additives, and certain foods.

Hodgkin's disease (HD)   A malignant disorder, usually arising in lymph nodes.

Human immunodeficiency virus (HIV)   The causative agent of AIDS. It is a retrovirus, which means that it carries its genetic information in RNA, and copies the genetic coding into DNA by using an enzyme called reverse transcriptase. The viral DNA is inserted into the host cell's DNA, and is used to produce more viruses.

Human leukocyte-associated antigens (HLAs)   Surface proteins on white blood cells and other nucleated cells that are unique for each person (except for identical twins) and are used to type tissues and help prevent rejection.

Hyaluronic acid   A viscous, amorphous extracellular material that binds cells together, lubricates joints, and maintains the shape of the eyeballs.

Hybridoma   A clone of cells produced by fusing a B cell with a tumor cell. This combines the B cell's ability to synthesize monoclonal antibody with the tumor cell's ability to grow indefinitely.

Hydrogen peroxide (H$_2$O$_2$)   A chemical produced by a phagocyte (inside the phagolysosome) that is highly destructive to the ingested particulate matter.

Hypersensitive   Allergic.

Hypersensitivity   Allergy.

IgA   The class of antibodies secreted by the lining of the body's various tracts (gastrointestinal, respiratory, urinary, and reproductive).

IgD   A class of antibodies; function unknown.

IgE   The class of antibodies that mediates Type I hypersensitive reactions and resistance to parasites.

IgG   The most abundant class of antibodies.

IgM   The class of antibodies that (along with IgG) provides most of the antibody-mediated immunity against bacteria and viruses.

Ileum   The terminal portion of the small intestine.

Immune adherence   *See* Opsonization.

Immune response   Altered reactivity to a specific microbe or foreign material that develops following contact with it. There are two basic types of immune responses: cell-mediated immunity (CMI) and antibody-mediated immunity (AMI). Most immune responses involve the interplay of both CMI and AMI. Also called a *specific response*.

Immunity   The state of being resistant to injury, particularly by poisons, foreign proteins, and invading pathogens.

Immunocompetence   The ability of B cells or T cells to carry out immune responses if properly stimulated.

Immunodeficiency   The absence of B cells or T cells. In combined immunodeficiency, both B cells and T cells are absent.

Immunogen   An antigen that elicits immunity.

Immunogenic   An antigen is said to be immunogenic if the response to the antigen leads to a state of immunity.

Immunogenicity   Ability of an antigen to stimulate immune responses.

Immunoglobulin (Ig)   A synonym for antibody. Immunoglobulins are divided into five clases : IgG, IgM, IgA, IgD, and IgE.

Immunological surveillance   The recognition and destruction of cancer (tumor) cells by cytotoxic T cells, macrophages, and natural killer cells. It is most effective in eliminating tumor cells that arise due to a cancer-causing virus. Also called *immune surveillance*.

Immunological tolerance   Lack of responsiveness (or hyporesponsiveness) to a particular antigen.

Immunology   The branch of science that deals with the responses of the body when challenged by antigens.

Immunosuppression   Inhibition of the immune response.

Immunotherapy   Attempt to induce the immune system to mount an attack against cancer cells.

Implantation   The insertion of a tissue or a part into the body.

Infection   Invasion and multiplication of microorganisms in body tissues, which may be inapparent or characterized by cellular injury.

Inflammation   Localized, protective response to tissue injury designed to destroy, dilute, or wall off the infecting agent or injured tissue. Characterized by redness, pain, heat, swelling, and sometimes loss of function. Also called the *inflammatory response*.

Ingestion   During phagocytosis, ingestion refers to the process by which a microbe is engulfed by a phagocyte. The plasma membrane of the phagocyte extends projections called pseudopods that surround the microbe, meet, and fuse, forming a membrane-enclosed sac called a phagosome.

Interferons (IFNs)   Antimicrobial substances produced by virus-infected lymphocytes, macrophages, and fibroblasts. Released IFNs diffuse to uninfected neighboring cells and bind to surface receptors, inducing the synthesis of proteins that inhibit viral replication. IFNs also suppress tumor formation and enhance the cell-killing activities of NK cells and phagocytes.

Interleukin-1 (IL-1)   A cytokine secreted by macrophages and other cells that acts as a costimulator during the activation of T cells and B cells.

Interleukin-2 (IL-2)   A cytokine secreted by activated helper T cells; it stimulates helper T cells, cytotoxic T cells, and NK cells to proliferate (multiply).

Interleukin-4 (IL-4)   A cytokine secreted by activated helper T cells that acts as a costimulator for B cells and causes plasma cells to secrete IgE antibodies.

Interleukin-5 (IL-5)   A cytokine secreted by activated CD4+T cells and mast cells that acts as a costimulator for B cells and causes plasma cells to secrete IgA antibodies.

Interstitial fluid   The fluid surrounding tissue cells. It is formed by the filtration of blood plasma into the tissue spaces and consists of blood plasma minus almost all of the plasma proteins, which pass through the capillary pores with difficulty. Every day about 3 liters of excess interstitial fluid is drained by lymphatic vessels and returned to the blood via the subclavian veins. After the interstitial fluid passes into the lymphatic vessels it is called lymph. Also called *tissue fluid*.

Keratinized cells   Flat, dead cells completely filled with a protein called keratin, forming the outermost layer of the skin epidermis. They form a physical barrier that protects the deeper tissues from microbial invasion, abrasion, and dehydration.

Kinins   Peptides that induce vasodilation of arterioles and increased permeability of capillaries near the site of infection or tissue damage; they also attract phagocytes to the site (act as chemotactic agents) and stimulate pain receptors. During inflammation, kinins are split from a plasma protein called kininogen.

Kupffer cell   *See* Stellate reticuloendothelial cell.

Lacrimal apparatus   A group of structures in the region of the eyes that produces and drains tears. Secretions of tears is a protective mechanism to dilute and wash away irritating substances and microbes. Blinking spreads tears over the surface of the eyeball.

Langerhans cell   Dendritic cells found in the skin epidermis. They trap antigens on their surfaces, then migrate to nearby lymph nodes, where they present the antigens (associated with MHC-II proteins) to helper T cells.

Lamina propria   The connective tissue layer of a mucous membrane. It contains diffuse lymphatic tissue (lymphatic tissue not enclosed by a capsule).

Left lymphatic duct   *See* Thoracic duct.

Leukemia   A malignant disease of the blood-forming tissues. Acute leukemia is characterized by uncontrolled production and accumulation of immature leukocytes. Chronic leukemia is characterized by an accumulation of mature leukocytes in the blood; the leukocytes do not die at the end of their normal life span.

Leukocyte   There are five types of leukocytes: neutrophils, eosinophils, basophils, lymphocytes, and monocytes. Also called a *white blood cell (WBC)*.

Leukocytosis   An increase in the production and release of white blood cells from bone marrow. Characteristic of many infections and other disorders. During inflammation, leukocytosis ensures a steady stream of neutrophils.

Leukopenia   A decrease in the number of white blood cells below 5,000/mm^3.

Leukotrienes (LTs)   Cytokines that function as mediators of inflammation.

Lumen   The space within an artery, vein, intestine, or a tube.

Lymph   Fluid confined in lymphatic vessels. Every day about 3 liters of excess interstitial fluid is drained by lymphatic vessels and returned to the blood via the subclavian veins. After the interstitial fluid passes into the lymphatic vessels it is called lymph. Lymph flows from the tissues via lymphatic vessels to the subclavian veins, where it returns to the blood. Any proteins that escape from blood capillaries during filtration cannot return to the blood by diffusion (the concentration gradient prevents it); lymphatic vessels return the leaked plasma proteins to the blood.

Lymphatic capillary   Closed-ended microscopic vessel that begins in the spaces between the cells and converges with other lymphatic capillaries to form lymphatic vessels.

Lymphatic nodules   Oval-shaped concentrations of lymphatic tissue not surrounded by a capsule. Most nodules are solitary, small, and discrete; they are scattered in the connective tissue layer (lamina propria) of mucous membranes. Some nodules occur in large, multiple aggregations in specific parts of the body; examples include the tonsils, Peyer's patches, and the vermiform appendix.

Lymphatic organs   Bone marrow, thymus gland, lymph nodes, and spleen.

Lymphatic system   The structural components of the lymphatic system include lymph, lymphatic vessels, and lymphatic tissues and organs. Its functions include protection against foreign invaders (immune responses), transport of lipids and fat-soluble vitamins, return of excess interstitial fluid to the blood, and return of plasma proteins to the blood.

Lymphatic tissue   A specialized form of reticular connective tissue that contains large numbers of lymphocytes. Also called *lymphoid tissue*.

Lymphatic vessel   A large vessel that collects lymph from lymphatic capillaries and converges with other lymphatic vessels to form lymph trunks. Structurally a lymphatic vessel resembles a vein, but it has thinner walls and more valves.

Lymph node   An oval or bean-shaped structure located along lymphatic vessels. It contains macrophages, dendritic cells, plasma cells, and lymphocytes.

Lymphocyte   The type of leukocyte (white blood cell) responsible for specific (immune) responses. There are two basic types of lymphocytes: B cells and T cells.

Lymphocyte activation   The proliferation (cell division by mitosis) and differentiation of B cell or T cells. B cells are differentiated into plasma cells and memory B cells; T cells are differentiated into cytotoxic T cells and memory T cells.

Lymphokines   Proteins secreted by lymphocytes. An example is interleukin-2 (IL-2), a substance secreted by activated T cells.

Lymphotoxin (LT)   A cytokine released by activated

cytotoxic T cells that kills target cells by causing the fragmentation of DNA.

Lymph trunks Lymphatic vessels unite to form larger tubes called lymph trunks. The principal lymph trunks are the right and left lumbar trunks, the intestinal trunk, the right and left bronchomediastinal trunks, the right and left subclavian trunks, and the right and left jugular trunks. They pass their lymph into the blood stream through the thoracic duct and the right lymphatic duct.

Lysis *See* Cytolysis.

Lysosome An organelle in the cytoplasm of a cell, enclosed by a single membrane and containing powerful digestive enzymes.

Lysozyme A bactericidal enzyme found in tears, saliva, and perspiration.

Macrophage Phagocytic cell derived from a monocyte. There are two basic types : fixed macrophages and wandering macrophages. Large numbers of macrophages are found in the lymph nodes, spleen, skin, liver, lungs. During cell-mediated immune responses, the secretion of lymphokines by activated T cells attracts macrophages to the site of infection. During antibody-mediated immune responses, macrophages ingest microbes coated with antibodies. Macrophages are probably involved in the response to malignant tumors, the rejection of allografts, and delayed-type hypersensitivity. In summary, they function as phagocytes and antigen presenting cells; they also secrete monokines involved in inflammation and the costimulation of lymphocytes.

Major histocompatibility complex antigens (MHC antigens) Several hundred thousand different glycoproteins that mark the surface of body cells. Their main function is to help T cells recognize foreign invaders. T cells can only recognize antigenic fragments that have first been processed and presented in association with MHC antigens. There are two categories : class I MHC antigens are expressed (displayed) on the surface of all body cells except red blood cells; class II MHC antigens are expressed on the surface of antigen presenting cells (dendritic cells, B cells, and some macrophages) and other cells involved in immune responses. Transplanted tissues are rejected because of incompatible MHC antigens. Also called *HLA antigen*.

Margination Accumulation and adhesion of neutrophils to the inner lining of blood capillaries at the site of injury; occurs during the early stages of inflammation.

Mast cell A cell found in the areolar connective tissue along blood vessels that produces heparin and histamine, which cause vasodilation during inflammation. A cell type derived from basophils.

Mediate Bring about.

Medulla The innermost portion of an organ; the opposite of cortex.

Membrane attack complex (MAC) A group of complement proteins (C5b, C6, C7, C8, and C9) that directly kills a microbe by forming channels in the plasma membrane, causing the microbe to rupture (cytolysis).

Memory One of the two main criteria for an immune response (the other is specificity). Memory refers to the fact that the second and subsequent responses to an agent are faster and more vigorous than the initial response.

Memory cell B cell or T cell that differentiates during an initial exposure to an antigen. During second and subsequent exposure to the same antigen, it responds rapidly and vigorously.

Microbe A microscopic organism. Bacterium, virus, fungus, or other parasite. Also called a *microorganism*.

Microglia Cells in the brain that carry on phagocytosis. Also called *brain macrophages*.

Microphage Granular leukocyte that carries on phagocytosis; especially neutrophils and eosinophils.

Migration The movement of phagocytes (neutrophils, macrophages, eosinophils, and monocytes) toward the site of an infection.

Mitosis The process in cell division by which DNA is duplicated and an identical set of chromosomes is acquired by each daughter cell.

Monoclonal antibody (MAb) Antibody produced by clones of B cells hybridized with cancerous cells.

Monocyte A type of leukocyte (white blood cell) that leaves the blood stream and is transformed into a macrophage.

Monokines Chemicals secreted by monocytes and macrophages. Monokines and lymphokines (secreted by lymphocytes) are collectively referred to as cytokines.

Mononuclear phagocytic system The combination of wandering macrophages and fixed macrophages. Wandering macrophages circulate in the blood and migrate to infected areas. Fixed macrophages reside in certain tissues and organs; especially the skin, liver, lungs, brain, bone marrow, lymph nodes, and spleen. Also called the *reticuloendothelial system*.

Mucous membrane A membrane that consists of an epithelial layer and an underlying connective tissue layer (the lamina propria). Mucous membranes line the gastrointestinal, respiratory, urinary and reproductive tracts. The epithelial layer secretes a sticky fluid called mucus, which traps many microbes and foreign substances. Mucous membranes in the nasal cavities have mucus-coated hairs that trap microbes, dust, and pollutants in the air; mucous membranes of the upper respiratory tract have cilia that propel the mucus up toward the throat, where it is swallowed. Penetration of the mucous membrane by microbes may be aided by mucosal irritations, toxins produced by microbes, and tissue injury resulting from viral infections. Also called the *mucosa*.

Mucus The thick fluid secrtion of mucous glands and mucous membranes.

Mutation Any change in the sequence of bases in the DNA molecule resulting in a permanent alteration in some inheritable characteristic.

Natural immunity The lack of susceptibility of humans to many animal diseases.

Natural killer cell (NK cell) Cells highly cytotoxic for tumor cells, but not for normal cells. Their action is nonspecific. Like cytotoxic T cells, they have cytoplasmic granules that contain perforin, a protein that forms holes in the plasma membranes of their target cells.

Necrosis Death of a cell or group of cells as a result of disease or injury.

Neutrophil One of the five basic types of white blood cells. A phagocytic cell, capable of ingesting and destroying particulate matter.

Nonspecific resistance Mechanisms that protect against the invasion of a broad range of microbes and foreign substances without having to recognize the specific agent. Nonspecific resistance involves physical and chemical barriers, inflammation, phagocytosis, antimicrobial substances, and natural killer cells.

Oncogene   Gene that has the ability to transform a normal cell into a cancerous cell when it is inappropriately activated. Oncogenes may be introduced into a cell by a retrovirus.

Oncology   The study of tumors.

Opsonin   The general name given to a chemical mediator that coats a microbe, enhancing phagocytosis.

Opsonization   The action of some antibodies and the C3b component of the complement system that renders bacteria and other foreign cells more susceptible to phagocytosis. Also called *immune adherence*.

Organism   Any living thing, single-celled or multicellular.

Oxidants   Lethal chemicals formed by phagocytes in a process called the respiratory (oxidative) burst. Examples include hydrogen peroxide, hypochlorite anion, and superoxide anion. They help kill phagocytized microbes.

Paracrine   Local hormone, such as histamine, that acts on neighboring cells.

Parasite   A disease-causing organsim.

Pathogen   A disease-causing organism.

Pathogenesis   The development of a disease; a morbid or pathological state.

Pathological   Pertaining to or caused by disease.

Perforin   A cytokine secreted by cytotoxic T cells and NK cells that forms channels in the plasma membrane of a target cell, causing it to rupture (cytolysis) and die.

Periarteriolar lymphatic sheath (PALS)   A layer of lymphatic tissue forming a sheath around a central artery in the spleen; consists mainly of T cells. Follicles, which are similar to the follicles in lymph nodes, are scattered throughout the PALS and consist of B cells.

Perspiration   Substance produced by sudoriferous (sweat) glands. Contains water, salts, urea, uric acid, amino acids, ammonia, sugar, lactic acid, and ascorbic acid.

Peyer's patches   Unencapsulated lymphatic nodules found in the lining of the small intestine. In the lower portion of the small intestine (ileum) there are about 30 patches, each consisting of 10 to 200 nodules.

Phagocyte   A cell capable of ingesting and destroying particulate matter, especially microbes and worn-out or damaged tissue cells. There are two major types of phagocytes: neutrophils and macrophages. Both neutrophils and macrophages express surface receptors for the Fc portion of IgG antibodies and the C3b fragment of complement. These receptors allow the phagocytes to bind antibody-coated targets and complement-coated targets, enhancing phagocytosis.

Phagocytic vesicle   *See* Phagosome.

Phagocytosis   The process by which cells (phagocytes) ingest particulate matter, especially microbes and worn-out or damaged tissue cells. The phagocytosis of some microbes can be greatly enhanced by coating the microbe surface with antibodies or C3b complement proteins.

Phagolysosome   The vesicle (membrane-enclosed sac) formed by the fusion of a phagosome and lysosome.

Phagolysosomes contain hydrolytic enzymes (lysozyme) and lethal oxidants (hydrogen peroxide), which break down microbial cell walls and degrade the macromolecules of the ingested material. Some microbes multiply within the phagolysosome and eventually destroy the phagocyte; an example is the *tubercle bacillus*. Some microbes, such as *staphylococci*, are not killed by phagocytosis; their toxins may kill the phagocyte. Other microbes, such as those that cause tularemia and brucellosis, may remain dormant in the phagolysosome for months or years.

Phagosome   A vesicle (membrane-enclosed sac) formed when a phagocyte engulfs particulate matter. Also called a *phagocytic vesicle*.

Pharynx   The throat.

Plasma   The extracellular fluid found in blood vessels; blood minus the formed elements.

Plasma cell   Cell that synthesizes and secretes antibodies. Activated B cells differentiate into plasma cells.

Plasma proteins   Proteins found the the blood plasma that are not used by cells (metabolized) for energy production, enzyme synthesis, or structural purposes. Albumins, globulins, and fibrinogen.

Pluripotent hematopoietic stem cell   Immature stem cell in bone marrow that gives rise to precursors of all the different mature blood cells. Previously called a *hemocytoblast*.

Present   During immune responses antigens are "presented" to lymphocytes (B cells or T cells). This means that the antigens are modified (processed) by a macrophage or dendritic cell and then inserted into their plasma membranes in a form that can be "recognized" by a lymphocyte. When "presented" in this fashion, the antigen can bind to a receptor on a lymphocyte, activating the lymphocyte.

Primary lymphatic organs   The primary lymphatic organs are the sites where lymphocytes mature (become immunocompetent cells). B cells mature in the red bone marrow; T cells mature in the thymus gland.

Primary response   The relatively slow response of the immune system after an initial contact with a particular antigen. The slow response is due to the fact that there are very few B cells or T cells that match the invading antigen and are able to respond. The proliferation and differentiation of the specific lymphocytes needed to attack the antigen may take several days.

Progeny   Refers to offspring or descendants.

Proliferation   Rapid and repeated reproduction of new cells.

Properdin   A protein found in serum capable of destroying bacteria and viruses.

Prostaglandins (PG)   A membrane-associated lipid composed of 20-carbon fatty acids with 5 carbon atoms joined to form a cyclopentane ring. During inflammation prostaglandins are released by damaged cells. They intensify the effects of histamine and kinins, which are also secreted and activated during inflammation.

Proto-oncogene   Gene responsible for some aspects of normal growth and development; it may transform into an oncogene, a gene capable of causing cancer.

Protozoa   (singular: protozoon)   One-celled animals.

Pus   The liquid product of inflammation. A collection of dead phagocytes, damaged tissue cells and fluid. Pus formation continues until an infection subsides.

Reactivity   Ability of an antigen to react specifically with the antibody whose formation it induced.

Recognition The binding of an antigen receptor on the surface of a B cell or T cell with its specific antigen. T cell receptors only recognize antigen that is associated with an MHC protein. B cell receptors can recognize unprocessed antigen in lymph or interstitial fluid or processed antigen that is *not* associated with MHC proteins.

Replication Duplication.

Residual bodies Structures in phagocytes that contain particulate matter that cannot be further degraded. Residual bodies migrate to the plasma membrane, fuse with it, and release their contents into the interstitial fluid by exocytosis.

Resistance Ability to ward off disease.

Respiratory burst The formation of lethal oxidants (hydrogen peroxide, superoxide anion, and hypochlorite anion) by a phagocytic cell during phagocytosis. Also called *oxidative burst*.

Reticular connective tissue A type of loose connective tissue characterized by the presence of reticular cells and reticular fibers. It is found in the liver, spleen, and lymph nodes. In lymphatic tissues, it provides a supporting framework for the lymphocytes.

Reticuloendothelial system *See* Mononuclear phagocytic system.

Retrovirus A type of virus that carries its genetic information in RNA, and copies the genetic coding into DNA by using an enzyme called reverse transcriptase.

Reverse transcriptase An enzyme present in a retrovirus that allows it to transcribe the genetic information coded in its RNA into DNA.

Right lymphatic duct A vessel of the lymphatic system that drains lymph from the upper right side of the body and empties it into the right subclavian vein.

Saliva A clear, alkaline, somewhat viscous secretion produced mostly by the three pairs of salivary glands. Contains various salts, mucin, lysozyme, amylase, and lipase. Saliva dilutes the numbers of microbes and washes them from the surfaces of the teeth and mucous membranes of the mouth, preventing colonization.

Sebaceous gland An exocrine gland in the dermis of the skin, almost always associated with a hair follicle; secretes sebum. Also called an *oil gland*.

Sebum Secretion of sebaceous (oil) glands.

Secondary lymphatic organs The lymph nodes and spleen; organs in which mature lymphocytes reside and become activated when stimulated by the appropriate antigens.

Secondary response Accelerated, more intense cell-mediated or antibody-mediated immune response on a subsequent exposure to an antigen after the initial exposure. The increased rate and intensity of the response is due to the fact that memory cells that are specific for the invading antigen already exist in the body. Usually the immune response is so fast and efficient that no symptoms occur.

Serum Plasma minus its clotting proteins.

Sinus (of a lymph node) An irregular space through which lymph percolates as it passes through a lymph node. The space just inside the capsule is called the subcapsular sinus; the spaces between the trabeculae and the lymphatic nodules are called the peritrabecular sinuses.

Sinusoid A microscopic space or passage for blood in certain organs such as the liver or spleen.

Specificity One of the two main criteria for an immune response (the other is memory). The ability of an antibody or T cell to distinguish between two different antigens. The altered response occurs only to the same antigen encountered before.

Specific response A response that depends on the recognition of specific microbes or foreign substances. There are two basic types of specific responses: antibody-mediated immunity (mediated by antibodies) and cell-mediated immunity (mediated by T cells). Also called an *immune response*.

Spleen Large mass of lymphatic tissue between the stomach and the diaphragm. Functions include phagocytosis, production of lymphocytes, and blood storage.

Splenic cords The cells between the sinusoids in the red pulp of the spleen. Includes reticular cells, macrophages, monocytes, lymphocytes, plasma cells, granulocytes, red blood cells, and platelets. Also called *Billroth's cords*.

Splenic nodule *See* Follicle.

Splenic pulp The tissue inside the spleen. There are two types of splenic pulp: white pulp and red pulp. The white pulp is mainly composed of lymphocytes, arranged around central arteries. In some areas of white pulp, lymphocytes are thickened into lymphatic nodules called splenic nodules. The red pulp contains many blood-filled spaces (sinusoids) and many types of cells arranged in cords (splenic cords). Also called the *parenchyma*.

Stellate reticuloendothelial cell Phagocytic cell found in liver sinusoids. Also called a *Kupffer's cell*.

Sudoriferous gland An apocrine or eccrine exocrine gland in the dermis or subcutaneous layer that produces perspiration. Also called a *sweat gland*.

Suppressor T cell (Ts cell) A class of T cell that inhibits antibody production and cytotoxic T cell activity.

Susceptibility Lack of resistance to the effects of pathogenic organisms.

T cell A lymphocyte that can differentiate into one of four kinds of cells: helper T cells, cytotoxic T cells, suppressor T cells, and memory T cells. Also called *T lymphocytes*.

T cell receptor (TCR) A protein on the surface of a T cell that recognizes (binds to) a specific antigen.

T lymphocytes Also called T cells.

Thoracic duct A lymphatic vessel that receives lymph from the left side of the head, neck, and chest, the left arm, and the entire body below the ribs, and empties into the left subclavian vein. Also called *left lymphatic duct*.

Thymus gland An organ with two lobes, located in the upper mediastinum posterior to the sternum and between the lungs which plays an essential role in the immune mechanism of the body.

Tissue macrophage system General term that refers to wandering and fixed macrophages.

Tissue rejection Phenomenon by which the body recognizes the protein (HLA antigens) in transplanted tissues or organs as foreign and produces antibodies against them.

Tonsil An aggregation of large lymphatic nodules embedded in the mucous membrane lining the throat. There are three types of tonsils: pharnygeal, palatine, and lingual.

Toxic Pertaining to poison; poisonous.

Toxoid Bacterial toxin treated with formaldehyde to destroy its toxicity; it retains its ability to elicit antibodies.

Trabecula (plural: trabeculae)   Fibrous cord of connective tissue serving as supporting fiber by forming a septum extending into an organ from its wall or capsule.   The thymus gland and lymph nodes have trabeculae.

Transferrins   Iron-binding proteins found in the blood plasma and interstitial fluids.   They inhibit bacterial growth by reducing the amount of available iron.

Transfusion   Transfer of whole blood, blood components, or bone marrow directly into the bloodstream.

Transplantation   The replacement of injured or diseased tissues or organs with natural ones.

Tumor cell   Cancer cell.

Tumor antigens   Unusual proteins that are produced by genetically altered tumor cells.   They are inserted in the plasma membranes of the tumor cells associated with MHC-I proteins.

Tumor necrosis factor   A cytokine secreted mainly by macrophages that stimulates the accumulation of leukocytes at the site of inflammation, activates leukocytes to kill microbes, stimulates the synthesis of IL-1 by macrophages, induces endothelial cells and fibroblasts to synthesize colony-stimulating factors, exerts an antiviral effect on body cells, and induces fever.

Type I hypersensitivity reaction   An allergic response mediated by IgE antibodies on the surface of mast cells and basophils.   Anaphylactic reactions may be localized (eczema, hives, abdominal cramps, and diarrhea) or systemic (bronchial constriction due to a wasp sting).   Also called *anaphylaxis.*

Type II hypersensitivity reaction   An allergic response mediated by IgG or IgM.   The reaction of antibodies with antigens on the surface of blood cells or tissue cells usually leads to the activation of complement.   During incompatible blood transfusions, the response may damage cells by causing lysis.   Also called *cytotoxic hypersensitive reaction.*

Type III hypersensitivity reaction   An allergic response mediated by IgA or IgM antibodies, complement, and antigens that are not part of a host tissue cell.   Antigen-antibody complexes become trapped in the basement membrane under the endothelium of blood vessels.   Complement is activated, causing inflammation.   Conditions that result from this reaction include rheumatoid arthritis (RA), systemic erythematosus (SLE), and glomerulonephritis.   Also called *immune complex hypersensitivity reaction.*

Type IV hypersensitivity reaction   An allergic response mediated by T cells.   It is called delayed hypersensitivity because it takes several days to develop.   An example is the skin rash caused by poison ivy.   Also called a *cell-mediated hypersensitivity reaction* or *delayed type hypersensitivity (DTH) reaction..*

Vaginal secretions   Vaginal secretions cleanse the vagina, preventing microbial colonization.

Vasoconstriction   A decrease in blood vessel diameter due to contraction of smooth muscle in the vessel walls.

Vasodilation   An increase in blood vessel diameter due to relaxation of smooth muscle in the vessel walls.   During inflammation, the vasodilation of local arterioles increases blood flow to a site of infection or tissue damage.   Vasodilation is stimulated by many different chemicals released during inflammation (i.e., histamine, kinins, prostaglandins, and certain complement proteins).

Venule   A small vein that collects blood from capillaries and delivers it to veins.

Vermiform appendix   A twisted, coiled tube attached to the cecum (first portion of the ascending colon).   Also called the *appendix.*

Wandering macrophages   Phagocytic cell that develops from a monocyte, leaves the blood, and migrates to infected tissues.

Wart   Generally benign tumor of epithelial skin cells caused by a virus.

White blood cell (WBC)   *See* Leukocyte.

Bibliography

Curtis, Helena.   *Biology,* 3rd ed.
New York : Worth, 1979.

Dorland, William Alexander.   *Dorland's Illustrated Medical Dictionary,* 27th ed.
Philadelphia : W. B. Saunders, 1988.

Ganong, William F.   *Review of Medical Physiology*, 15th ed.
Norwalk, Connecticut : Appleton & Lange, 1991.

Junqueira, L. Carlos, Jose Carneiro, and Robert O. Kelley.   *Basic Histology*, 6th ed.
Norwalk, Connecticut : Appleton & Lange, 1989.

Kimball, John W.   *Biology*, 4th ed.
Reading, Massachusetts : Addison-Wesley, 1978.

Kimball, John W.   *Introduction to Immunology*, 3rd ed.
New York : Macmillan, 1990.

Melloni, B.J., Ida Dox, and Gilbert Eisner.   *Melloni's Illustrated Medical Dictionary*, 2nd ed.
Baltimore : Williams & Wilkins, 1992.

Roitt, Ivan, Johathan Brostoff, and David Male.   *Immunology*, 2nd ed.
London : Gower, 1989.

Tortora, Gerard J. and Sandra Reynolds Grabowski.   *Principles of Anatomy and Physiology,* 7th ed.
New York : HarperCollins, 1993.

Vander, Arthur J., James H. Sherman, and Dorothy S. Luciano.   *Human Physiology,* 5th ed.
New York : McGraw-Hill, 1990.